The Dash Diet for Beginners

Simple and Healthy Recipes for Every Meal

Martin Peters

Table of Contents

Introduction: Everything You Need to Know About the Dash Diet

The dash diet is not a new word around, as it is one of the proven diet plans that help maintain hypertension, reduce stress, and increase mental and physical health. This chapter deal with everything you need to know about the dash diet and the basic aim is to sever the purpose of making people aware of the diet plan. We hope that after reading this book you will get a better understanding of the diet, its history, pros, and cons along with 50 easy to prepare recipes that are delicious and helps you to control high blood pressure without sacrificing the taste. Now, let us look at the basic definition of the diet.

What Is DASH Diet? Basic definition

The dash diet is an approved diet plan that lowers hypertension by reducing salt intake. As we know that the salt is a key factor in making the blood pressure high. The high blood pressure if not addressed lead to kidney diseases, heart attack, and cirrhosis

The focus of this diet is on vegetables, fruits, white meat, and some nuts and seafood items. Low dairy products are allowed in this diet plan. There is a big no to artificial drinks, red meat, beverages, and junk. In the end, the intake of less salt in daily meal plans makes a huge difference.
 So, according to "Dietary Guidelines for Americans, 2010", the salt intake should not be more than 1500 mg on daily basis.

Who Can Follow A DASH Diet?

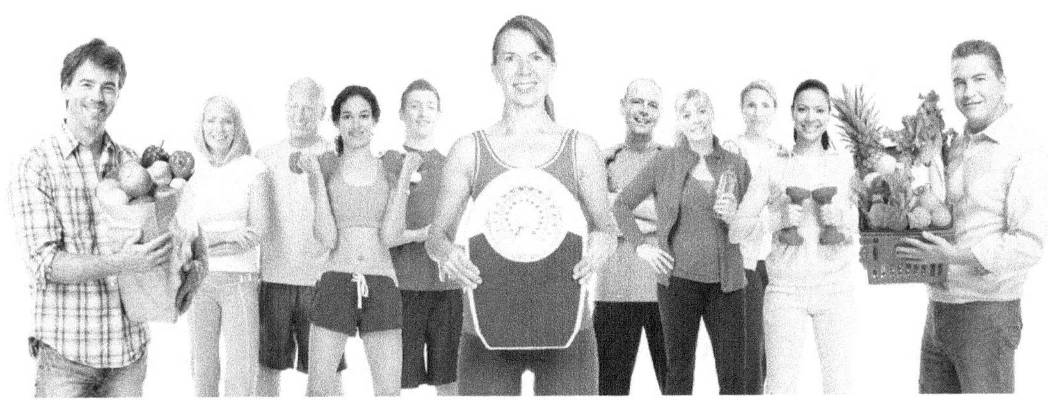

- It can be followed by people having kidney disease
- It is a perfect diet plan for people having hypertension
- It can also be followed by people with diabetes
- It is suited for American citizens
- It is suited for African citizens
- Old and middle-aged people can easily follow this diet plan

The advice that our parents and grandparent give us about eating a lot of veggies, fruits, and drinking milk on daily basis is something parallel to the DASH diet.

It is very important to indulge in healthy eating and include seasonal fruits and vegetables in the diet plan. The dash diet offers some herbs, condiments, and spices that are alternatives to salt like, vinegar, garlic, and lemon juice.

The Basic Goal of DASH Diet

The basic goal to achieve while following dash diet is based on 2000 calories plan that is well known as " Your Guide to Lowering Your Blood Pressure with DASH." The recommendations on daily basis are as followed:

- Sodium 2300 mg
- Saturated fat 6% of calories
- Total fat 27% of calories
- Potassium 4700 mg
- Calcium 1,250 mg
- Cholesterol 150 mg
- Protein 18% of calories
- Magnesium 500 mg
- Carbohydrates 55% of calories

When you decided to follow this diet plan then it is very curial to pick the best, organic, and seasonal food items that play a role in achieving the ratios that are defined above. When following a DASH diet, it is very important to pick the best ingredients that play a significant role in counting the intake of fat, protein, sodium, sugar, and potassium.

You just need to eliminate all those items that cause hypertension like broth, garlic, beans, and bouillons cubes.

The dash diet is the ultimate diet plan that makes you healthy and happy. If you want to transform your physical shape and mental health, or if you are aged between 19 to 55 then this diet is highly recommended for you to control hypertension and gain more health and fitness for the long term.

The   DASH diet offers 2000 calories a day, including:

- Fruit: 5-6 servings per day
- Sodium: 2,300 mg per day
- Vegetable 4 – 5 servings a day
- Meat, fish, and poultry <6 serving per day
- Low-fat dairy products: 2-3 servings per day
- Nuts, seeds, beans, peas: 4-5 serving for a full week.
- Grains: 6-8 servings each day
- Oils: 2-3 servings for one day
- Sweets: 5 servings for one week

DASH Diet _Addressing Hypertension

The terms hypertension and high blood pressure both are interlinked. So, if you are suffering from one of these you will feel no pain or symptoms. To get to know about it, you need to have a proper checkup. There are a lot of high blood pressure patients who also suffer from hypertension. Hypertension is serious and life-threatening. This is the reason hypertension is called a silent killer. The DASH diet is the only diet plan that focuses and reduces the symptom of both conditions.

Food Include and Eliminate in the DASH Diet

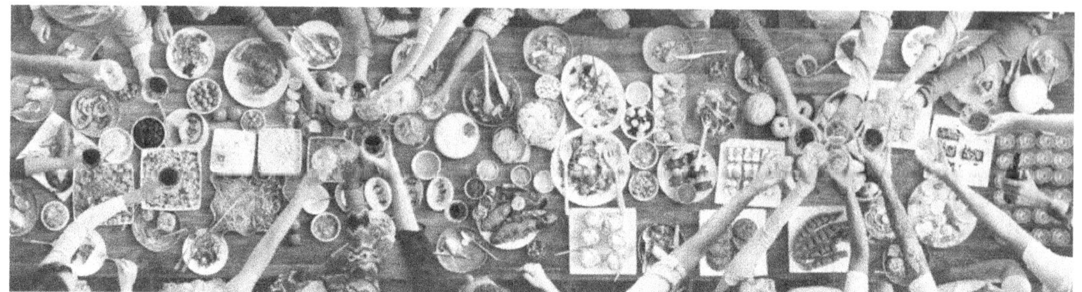

The low sodium diet plan forbids excess salt. Listed below is the list of food allowed and not allowed.

Food Allowed on the DASH diet

- Vegetables: mostly green leafy vegetables
- lean protein: like eggs, fish, turkey, chicken
- Fruits: like apple, orange, grapefruits, pineapple, berries, banana
- Grains: whole and unprocessed
- Nuts/nut oils: sunflower oil, olive oil
- Seeds, sunflower seeds, sesame seed
- Low-fat dairy products: low-fat cheese, low-fat mayonnaise
- Vegetable oils

Food to Avoid on a DASH diet plan

- Sweets
- Artificial flavors
- Beverage
- Canned sodas
- Canned juices
- Red meat
- Processed food items
- Artificial sugar

Advantages of a DASH Diet

- This diet plan effectively lowers cholesterol and hypertension.
- It helps improve mental health and improves mood.
- It eliminates and reduces the risks of kidney failure.
- This diet plan helps you to detoxify the body.
- The dash diet plan helps in cutting the fat and reducing some extra pounds.
- It reduces the risk of heart attack and its related illnesses.
- Helps lower blood pressure in a shorter period.

Tips and Cautions While Following a Dash Diet Plan

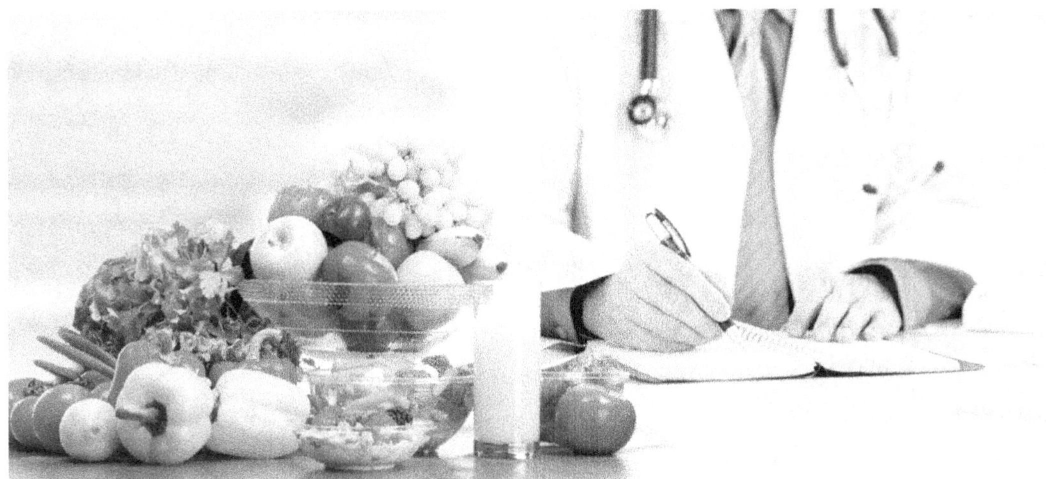

It is necessary to ask the doctor before starting a dash diet plan, though it is a safe diet still a lot of people are already following medications that help them lower hypertension. Moreover, individual needs are different so it might be required to stop or reduce the mediation that is been taken already.

With that keeping track of the blood pressure is also necessary. So, it is also recommended to have a proper professional check-up monthly.

It is crucial to note that the DASH diet works and affects different for everyone, for example, a person who has kidney disease may have a different effect of diet, than the person who does not have kidney disease. Sugar subtitles on the DASH diet plan

- Applesauce
- Orange juice
- Grape juice
- Dates
- Raisins
- Dry cranberries

Salt substitutes

- Ginger
- Rosemary
- Paprika
- Sage
- Dill
- Thyme
- lemon zest
- Lemon juice
- Lime juice
- Curry powder
- Cinnamon,
- Nutmeg
- Oregano
- Poorer
- Marjoram
- Cloves
- Sage
- Onion
- onion powder
- Parsley

- Garlic
- Bay leaf

The dash diet is a sustainable diet plan that helps you enjoy some delicious food, while keeping your blood pressure low. It is an effective diet plan to low sodium, fat, and sugar.
most of the highly processed and artificial flavored foods are discouraged in this diet plan. The main emphasis is on protein.

Pros Of DASH Diet Plan

It is easy to follow, a safe, and low-budgeted diet plan that has such ingredients that help you cure hunger pangs and sweet cravings. All the items allowed in the diet are accessible.

This diet plan is not like any marketing gambit that is costly and needs money to join an online course.

It is a very flexible plan having different calorie levels, including 1200, 1600, 2600, and 3100.

Depending on a person's gender and weight anyone starts the DASH diet right away.

Does the DASH diet help you lose weight?

You can enjoy its proven benefits, to make yourself active, stress-free, energetic, healthy, and active.
This diet plan is nutrient-dense that fulfills all the growing body requirements. The calories are low that makes weight loss possible. This diet plan is also endorsed by the American Heart Association and National Institutes of Health, USDA.

History of DASH Diet

in 1992, after examining the high ratio of people having hypertension, the American national institute of health addressed the disease and work toward some effective planning to lessen the effect of hypertension thus introduces a dietary pattern for all hypertension patients, which was named the DASH diet plan. Since then, people are following this effective plan that comes out of the NIH funding research.

If you are the one suffering from hypertension patient and do not want your health and condition to fade away, then you need to follow a DASH diet plan.

The next part of the cookbook deals with preparing some delicious dash diet recipes. So, if you are a busy housewife or a professional having on-the-go life and could not find time to prepare a meal that helps you reduce the symptoms of hypertension and high blood pressure way then stop worrying.

With a perceptive ingredient list and making a few adjustments to your eating habits, you can make some low sodium recipes in a few minutes

- We recommend reading complete recipes before starting the cooking process.
- Wash, cut, chop, prepare and set out all listed ingredients before cooking.
- Set out all necessary appliances and tools for cooking.
- Use a clean workplace and stove
- Try to incorporate organic and whole ingredients.
- Use vinegar, ginger instead of salt.

Now, let us start with the cooking.

10 breakfast Recipes

Spinach And Orange Bell Pepper Omelet

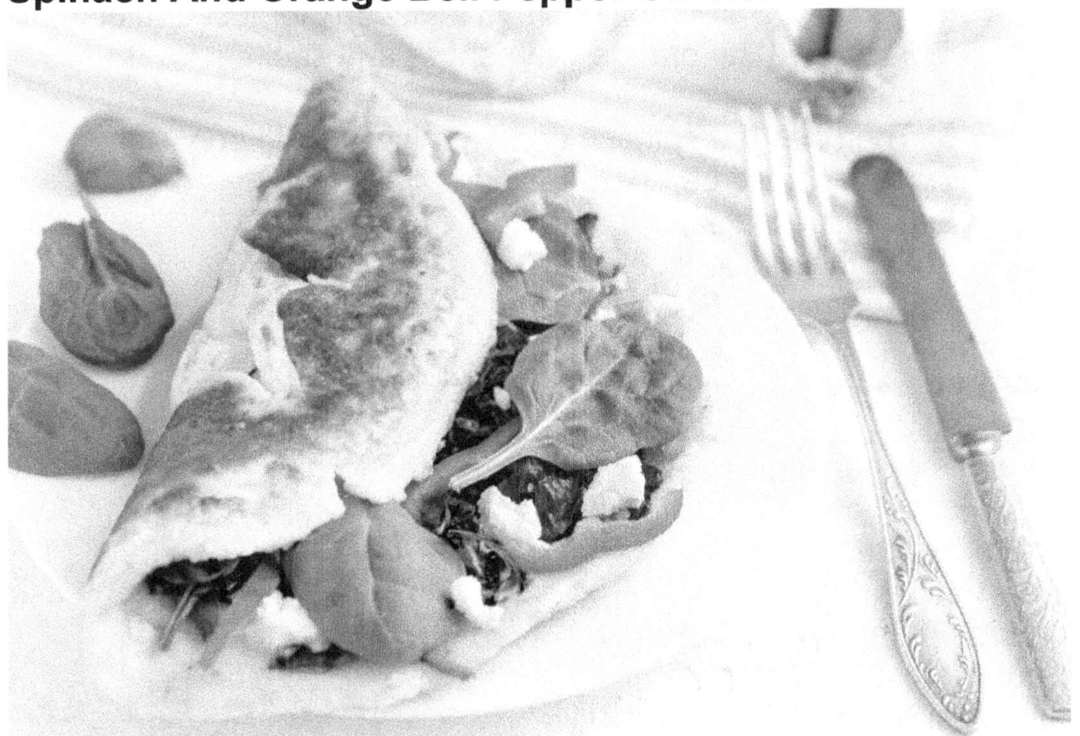

Preparation Time: 10 minutes
Cooking Time: 12 minutes
Servings: 2

Ingredients

- 2 teaspoons of olive oil
- 1 green onion, chopped
- ¼ cup of orange bell pepper, chopped
- 1 cup of spinach, thawed and chopped
- 1 cup egg whites, whisked
- Black pepper, to taste

Directions

1. The first step is to wash the spinach and remove its stem.
2. Thawed the spinach and then set it aside for further use.
3. Take a nonstick pan or skillet and heat olive oil in it.
4. Add in the green onions and let it cook for just a minute.
5. Then add the orange bell pepper and sauté it for 2 minutes
6. Then add the spinach and pour in whisked egg whites.
7. Heat should be low to medium.
8. Sprinkle black pepper on top.
9. Let the omelet cook until eggs get firm.
10. Serve it hot.

Nutrition Facts

Servings: 2
Amount per serving
Calories   114
% Daily Value*
Total Fat 5g   6%
Saturated Fat 0.7g   3%
Cholesterol 0mg 0%
Sodium 136mg   6%
Total Carbohydrate 3.1g   1%
Dietary Fiber 0.7g   3%
Total Sugars 1.8g
Protein 14g

Salmon and Eggs Scramble

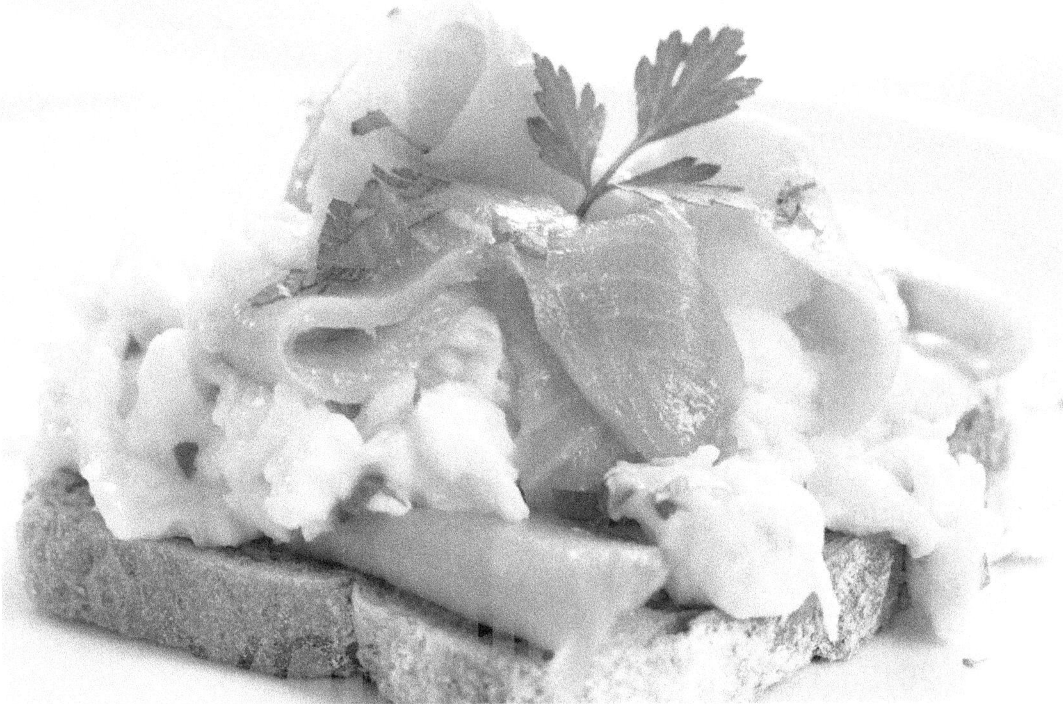

Preparation Time: 12 minutes
Cooking Time: 10 minutes
Servings: 2

Ingredients

- 2 teaspoons of vegetable oil
- 1 cup egg whites, whisked
- 2 tablespoons of low-fat milk
- ½ cup smoked salmon, crumbled
- 1/6 teaspoon of ginger and garlic paste
- ½ small white onion, chopped
- 2 slices of whole wheat bread, toasted

Directions

1. Take a skillet and heat oil in it.
2. Then saut é the onions in it for 2 minutes and add ginger and garlic paste.
3. Let it cook until the aroma comes.
4. Then whisk milk with egg whites and add in the crumbled salmon.
5. Pour it in the skillet and lower the heat
6. Let it cook unit the eggs get firm.
7. Serve hot with toasted whole wheat bread.

Nutrition Facts

Servings: 2

Amount per serving

Calories 335

% Daily Value*

Total Fat 11.4g 15%

Saturated Fat 2.4g 12%

Cholesterol 30mg 10%

Sodium 2812mg 122%

Total Carbohydrate 14.8g 5%

Dietary Fiber 2.3g 8%

Total Sugars 4g

Protein 40.9g

Pumpkin Muffins

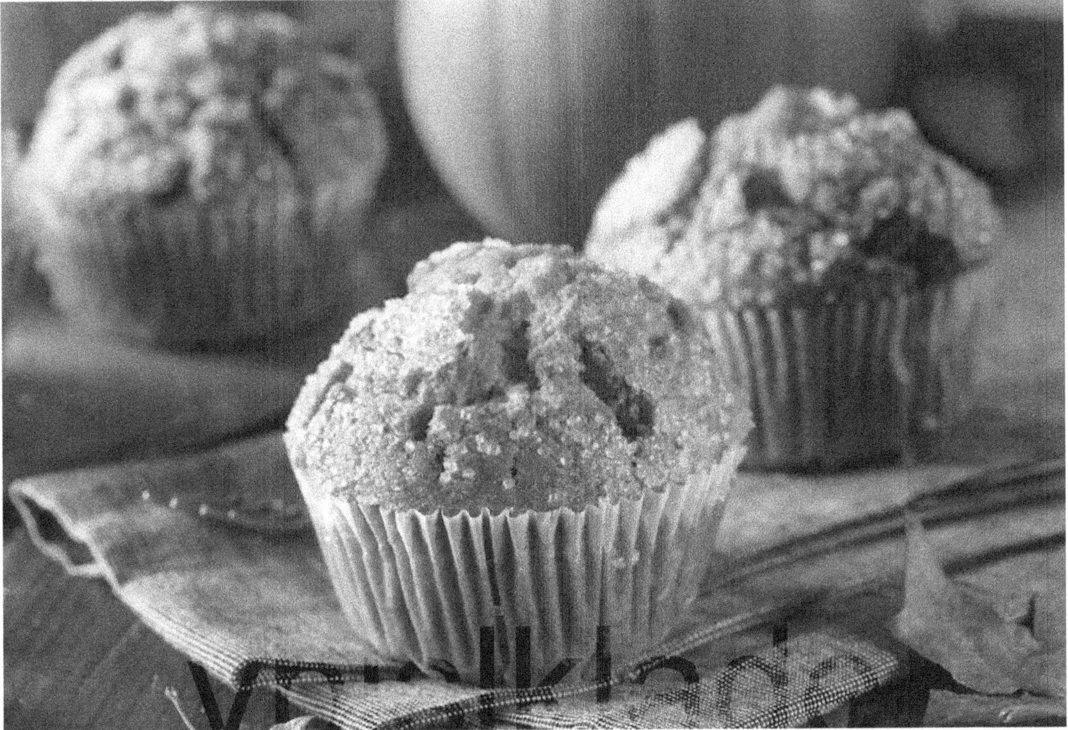

Preparation Time: 20minutes
Cooking Time: 55 minutes
Servings: 4
Ingredients

- 2 cups of almond flour
- 2 cups of pumpkin
- 4 large eggs
- 1 /2 teaspoon of baking powder
- ½ teaspoon of baking soda
- ¼ teaspoon of ground cinnamon
- 4 tablespoons of agave nectar
- 4 teaspoons almond butter
- Oil spray, for greasing

Directions

1. Preheat your oven to 360 degrees F.
2. Cube the pumpkin by peeling and taking out the seeds.
3. Cook it in the oven for about 30 minutes at 400 degrees F.
4. Take it out and puree it in a blender.
5. In a large bowl add the pumpkin puree, almond flour, baking powder, baking soda, and eggs, almond butter, agave nectar, and cinnamon.
6. Mix it well to form a batter.
7. Then pour the mixture into oil greased muffin tray.
8. Bake inside preheated oven for 25 minutes.
9. Once, golden from the top,
10. Serve and enjoy.

Nutrition Facts

Servings: 4

Amount per serving

Calories   293

% Daily Value*

Total Fat 21.5g   28%

Saturated Fat 3g 15%

Cholesterol 186mg   62%

Sodium 236mg   10%

Total Carbohydrate 16.7g   6%

Dietary Fiber 6.7g   24%

Total Sugars 5.6g

Protein 14.1g

Salmon Avocado Toast

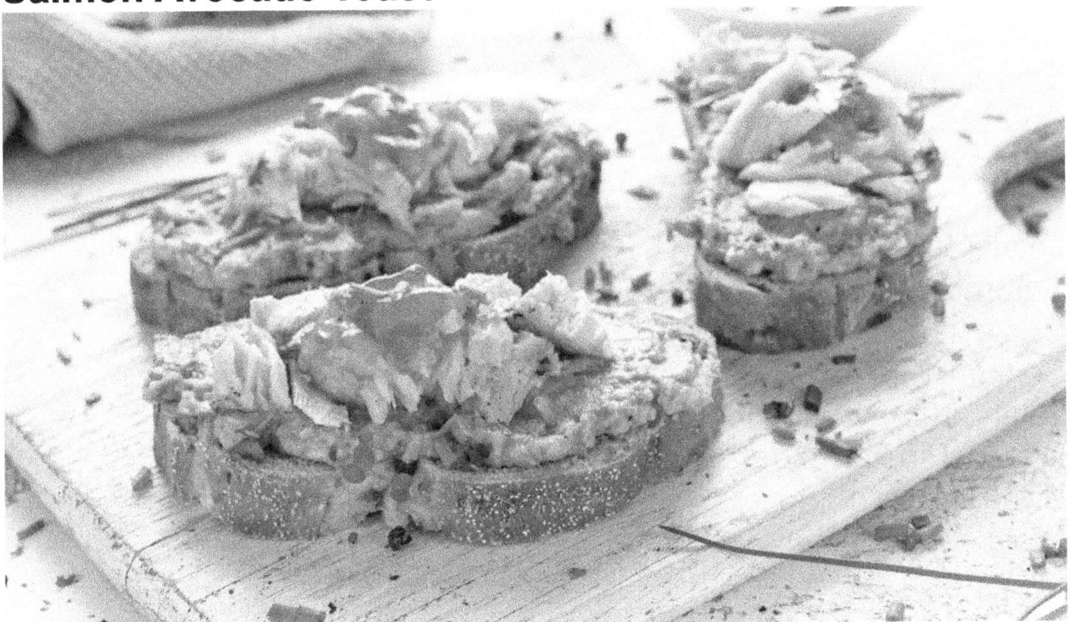

Preparation Time: 5 minutes
Cooking Time: 2 minutes
Servings: 2

Ingredients

- 4 slices Sprouted Whole Grain Bread
- 1 medium avocado
- 6 ounces of Smoked Salmon
- Pinch Salt-Free Garlic & Herb Seasoning

Directions

1. The first step is to toast the slices of bread in the toaster.
2. Then peel the avocado and layer it evenly over toast slices.
3. Top it with an equal number of salmon and sprinkle some salt-free garlic and herb seasoning

4. Enjoy

Nutrition Facts
Servings: 2
Amount per serving
Calories   465
% Daily Value*
Total Fat 23.3g   30%
Saturated Fat 4.9g   25%
Cholesterol 20mg   7%
Sodium 1837mg 80%
Total Carbohydrate 44.6g   16%
Dietary Fiber 10.7g   38%
Total Sugars 10.5g
Protein 23.5g

Overnight Oats

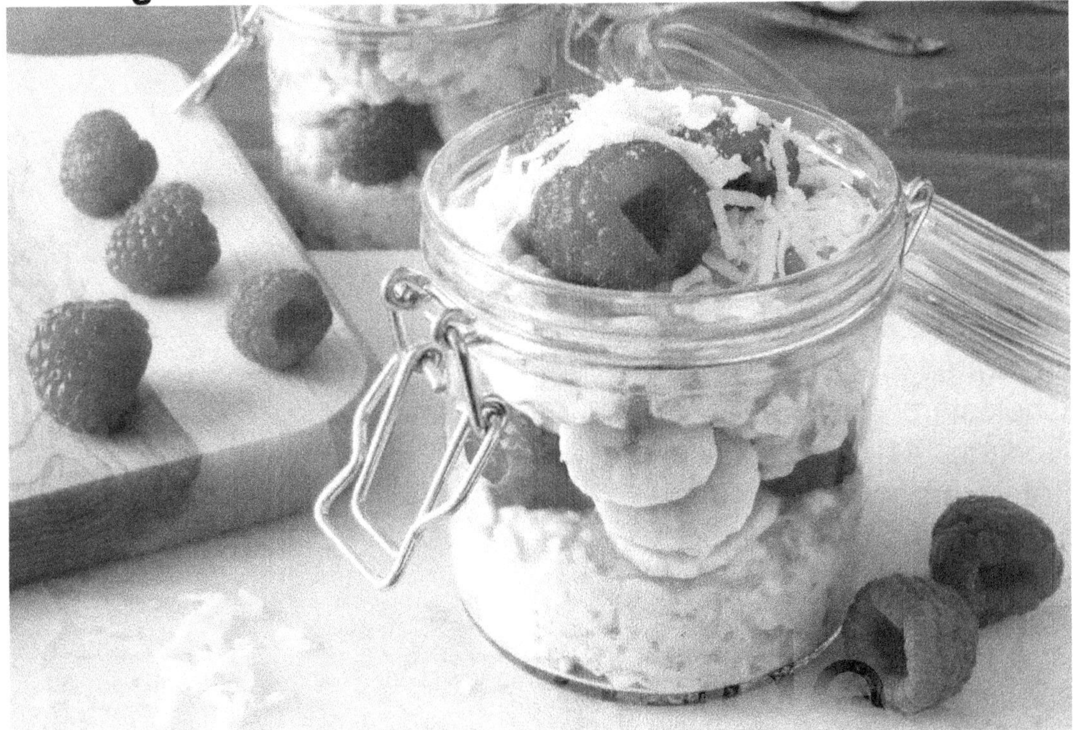

Preparation Time: 5 minutes
Cooking Time: minutes
Servings: 1
Ingredients

- 1/4 cup rolled oats
- 3/4 cup unsweetened almond milk
- 1/3 cup pumpkin puree
- 1/4 teaspoon cinnamon
- ¼ teaspoon pumpkin spice
- 1/4 teaspoon maple syrup
- 1 teaspoon pumpkin seeds

Directions

1. Combine all the listed ingredients in a mason jar.
2. Place it in refrigerators overnight.
3. Serve with the garnish of pumpkin seeds.

Nutrition Facts
Servings: 1
Amount per serving
Calories   158
% Daily Value*
Total Fat 5.6g   7%
Saturated Fat 0.9g   4%
Cholesterol 0mg 0%
Sodium 141mg   6%
Total Carbohydrate 24.4g   9%
Dietary Fiber 5.7g   20%
Total Sugars 4g
Protein 5.1g

Mushrooms and Eggs

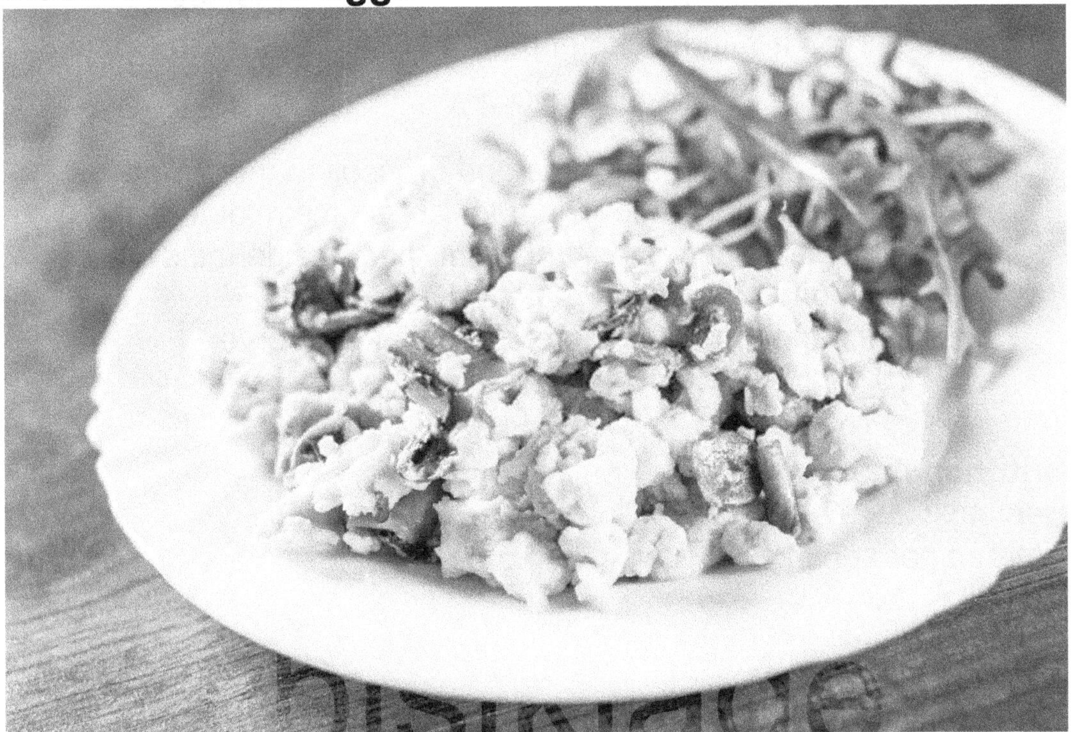

Preparation Time: 10minutes
Cooking Time: 15 minutes
Servings: 2

Ingredients

- 1 cup broccoli, thinly sliced
- 2 tablespoons of olive oil
- 4 organic eggs, whisked
- 2 medium onions, finely diced
- 10 wild mushrooms, finely chopped
- Black pepper to taste
- Pinch Salt-Free Garlic & Herb Seasoning
- 2 tomatoes, chopped

Directions

1. Take a nonstick skillet and heat oil in it
2. Then saut é the onions and add in the tomatoes.
3. season it with black pepper and Pinch Salt-Free Garlic & Herb Seasoning
4. cook it for 2 minutes.
5. then add the mushrooms and broccoli to the skillet.
6. and let it cook on low heat for about five minutes.
7. Whisk eggs in a bowl and pour them inside the skillet.
8. cook until the omelet gets firm.
9. Once the omelet is thoroughly cooked, serve.
10.	Enjoy.

Nutrition Facts
Servings: 2
Amount per serving
Calories   347
% Daily Value*
Total Fat 23.5g   30%
Saturated Fat 4.8g   24%
Cholesterol 327mg   109%
Sodium 154mg   7%
Total Carbohydrate 21.7g   8%
Dietary Fiber 5.9g   21%
Total Sugars 10.9g
Protein 17.5g

Sweet Potato Hash Browns

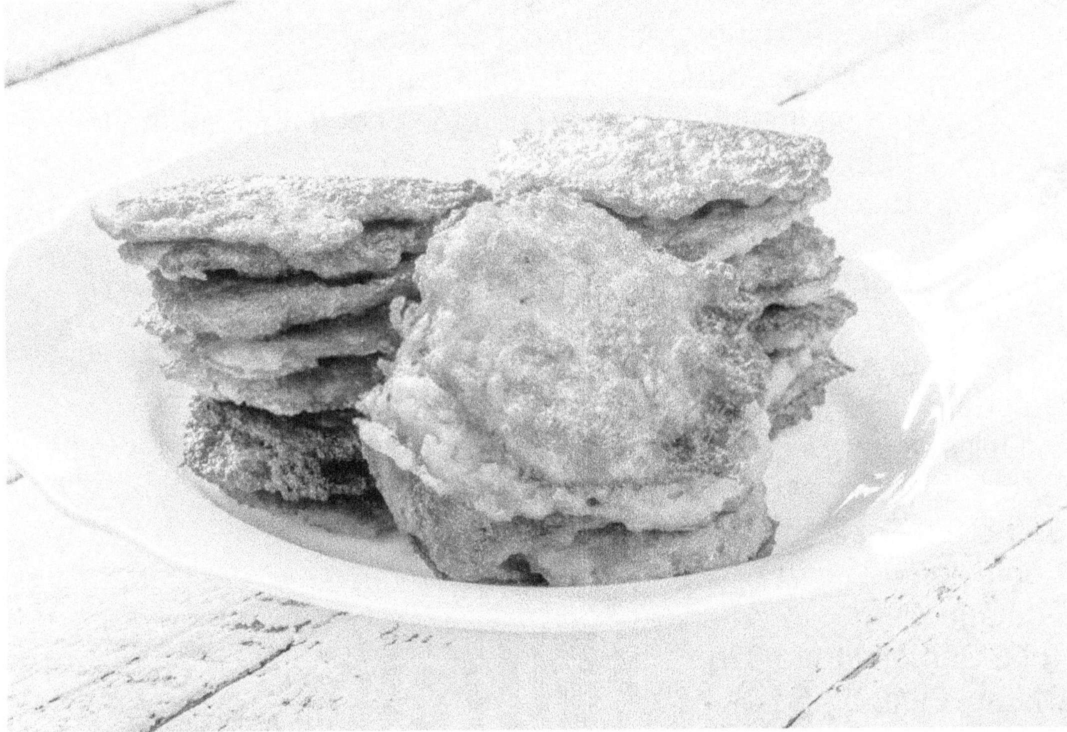

Preparation Time: 12 minutes
Cooking Time: 15 minutes
Servings: 2

Ingredients

- 4 large, sweet potatoes, peeled and grated
- 2 tablespoons olive oil
- 1 cup onion, chopped
- ¼ teaspoon Garlic & Herb Seasoning
- Black pepper to taste

Directions

1. Take a skillet and heat oil in it.

2. Saut é chopped onions in it and season it with Garlic &
   Herb Seasoning and black pepper
3. Then add the grated sweet potatoes.
4. Cook the potatoes for 15 minutes, until soft.
5. put on the lid and let the potatoes cook until golden for
   both sides.
6. Enjoy.

Nutrition Facts
Servings: 2
Amount per serving
Calories   497
% Daily Value*
Total Fat 14.6g   19%
Saturated Fat 2.1g   11%
Cholesterol 0mg 0%
Sodium 42mg   2%
Total Carbohydrate 89g   32%
Dietary Fiber 13.5g   48%
Total Sugars 3.9g
Protein 5.2g

Walnut and Blue Berry Pancake

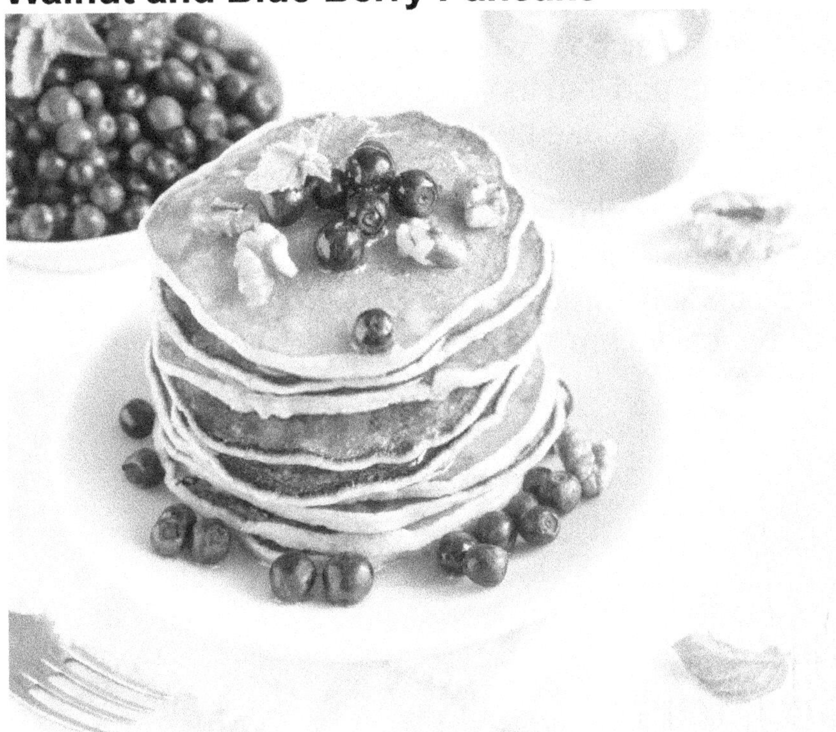

Preparation Time: 22 minutes
Cooking Time: 25 minutes
Servings: 4

Ingredients

- 2 cups of almond flour
- 2 organic eggs
- 2 teaspoons of walnut oil
- 1/3 cup of chopped walnuts
- 1 cup of blueberries
- 1 teaspoon baking powder
- Honey, topping (optional)

Directions

1. Take a large bowl and combine the almond flour, baking powder, and chopped walnuts.
2. In a separate small bowl whisk eggs and add in the oil.
3. beat it well and add it to the flour mixture
4. combine it to a pancake batter and fold in the blueberries
5. mix it well.
6. take a large pan and mist it with oil spray.
7. pour the spoonful on it.
8. Once the bubbles formed, flip to cook from the other side.
9. Once all pancakes are done, serve and enjoy with a drizzle of honey.

Nutrition Facts

Servings: 4

Amount per serving

Calories   143

% Daily Value*

Total Fat 10.1g   13%

Saturated Fat 1.3g   6%

Cholesterol 82mg   27%

Sodium 32mg   1%

Total Carbohydrate 9.2g   3%

Dietary Fiber 2.5g   9%

Total Sugars 4.4g

Protein 6.4g

Raspberry Smoothie

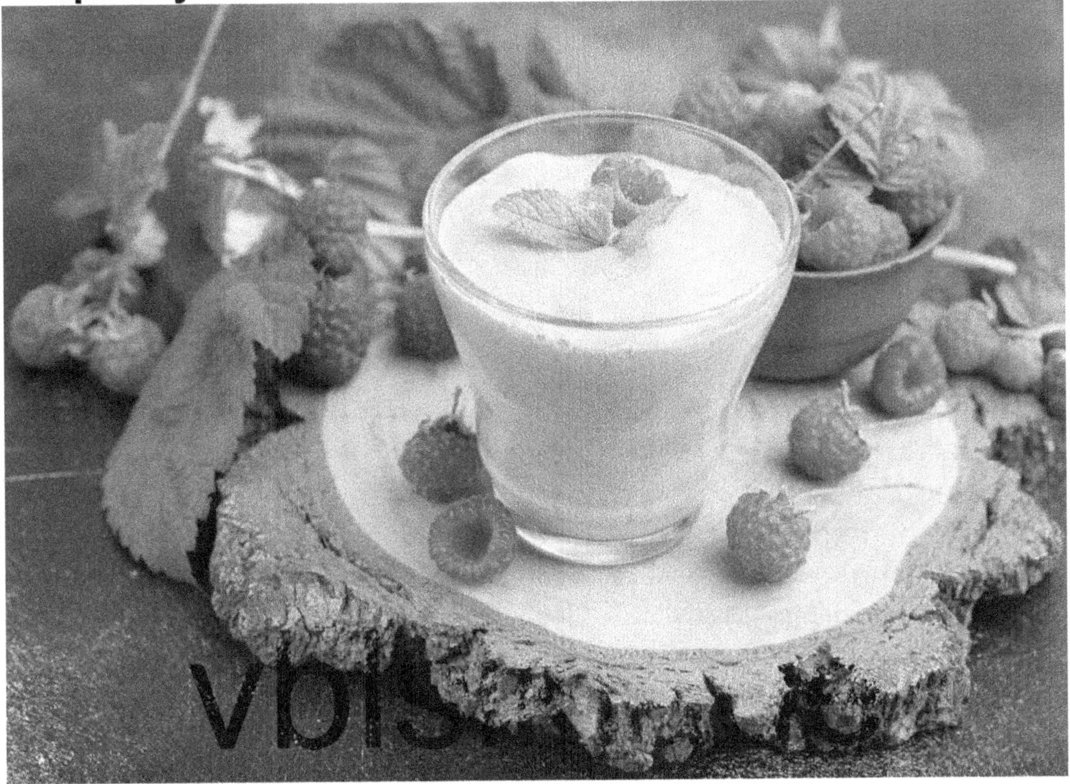

Preparation Time: 5 minutes
Cooking Time: 0 minutes
Servings: 2

Ingredients

- 1 cup baby spinach, chop
- 2 cups raspberries, fresh
- A ½ Tomato
- 2 cups of water
- 1 cup strawberries
- Few ice cubes, for chilling

Directions

1. First, you need to wash all the fruits and vegetables and remove the stems of spinach.
2. add all the listed ingredients into a high-speed blender.
3. pulse it until smooth.
4. pour into tall serving glasses and enjoy.
5. best served chilled.

Nutrition Facts
Servings: 2
Amount per serving
Calories   90
% Daily Value*
Total Fat 1.1g   1%
Saturated Fat 0g 0%
Cholesterol 0mg 0%
Sodium 21mg   1%
Total Carbohydrate 20.8g   8%
Dietary Fiber 9.8g   35%
Total Sugars 9g
Protein 2.4g

Healthy Breakfast Burrito

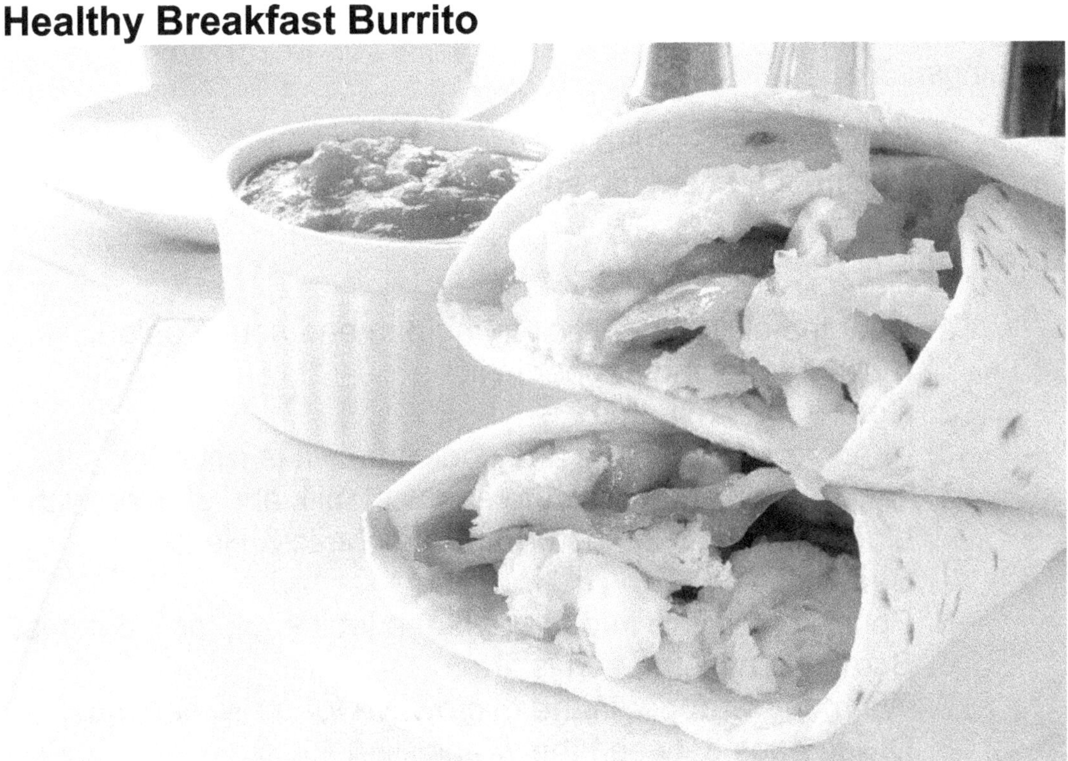

Preparation Time: 15 minutes
Cooking Time: 20 minutes
Servings: 4

Ingredients

- 4 Sprouted Wraps/Tortillas
- 8 large eggs
- ½ cup of low-fat milk
- 2 tablespoons olive oil
- 1/4 cups of onions, chopped
- ½ red pepper, chopped
- ½ cups mushrooms, sliced
- 2 cups baby spinach
- Black pepper, to taste

- Pinch of Salt-Free Garlic & Herb Seasoning

Toppings:

- 6 tablespoons sharp cheese (Cortijo)
- ¼ cup of homemade salsa

Directions

1. Heat the oil in a nonstick frying pan and saut é onion, mushrooms, and pepper in it.
2. Cook it for 3 minutes.
3. Then add the spinach and cook it until it is wilted.
4. Take a bowl and whisk the egg with milk and season with black pepper and Pinch Salt-Free Garlic & Herb Seasoning.
5. Pour egg mixture into the pan and let it cook for 3-6 mites.
6. Scramble until the egg is firm.
7. Warm the wrapper in the microwave for a few seconds.
8. Divide eggs between the wraps.
9. Sprinkle each burrito with cheese and homemade salsa.
10. Wrap up and enjoy a delicious breakfast.

Nutrition Facts

Servings: 4
Amount per serving
Calories   253
% Daily Value*
Total Fat 19.6g   25%
Saturated Fat 5.8g   29%
Cholesterol 381mg   127%
Sodium 200mg   9%
Total Carbohydrate 4.7g   2%
Dietary Fiber 0.5g   2%
Total Sugars 3.6g

Protein 15.9g

10 Lunch Recipes

Lentil Soup

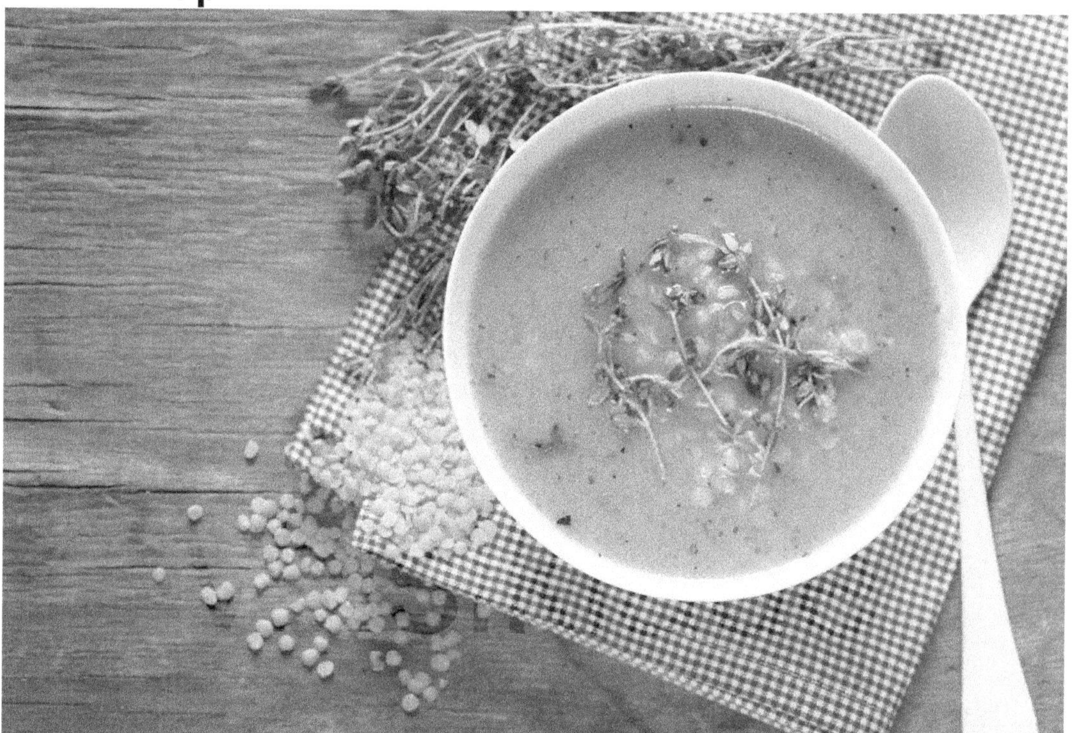

Preparation Time: 20 minutes
Cooking Time: 35 minutes
Servings: 4

Ingredients

- 2 tablespoons vegetable oil
- 1 green onion, chopped
- 2 teaspoons of garlic
- ½ teaspoon of ginger, chopped
- 6 plum tomatoes, chopped
- 3 cups apricots

- 1 cup of mushrooms, chopped
- 1 cup red lentils, rinsed
- 8 cups water
- 1 teaspoon of curry powder
- 1 cup coconut milk
- Black pepper, to taste

Directions

1. take a cooking pot and heat oil to saut é green onion.
2. Then add garlic, ginger, black pepper, and curry powder.
3. cook until aroma comes.
4. next add the dry apricots, water, tomatoes, mushrooms, and red lentils.
5. Cook on high heat for about 8 minutes.
6. next, lower the heat and cook for15 minutes with the lid on top.
7. Once, the lentils get soft, turn off the heat.
8. Let it get cool.
9. Pour the soup into the blender.
10. Transfer the soup back to the pan.
11. Let it simmer for 15 minutes and then add in the coconut milk.
12. Let it cook for 5 more minutes unit thickened.
13. Serve and enjoy hot.

Nutrition Facts

Servings: 4
Amount per serving
Calories   475
% Daily Value*
Total Fat 22.9g   29%
Saturated Fat 14.2g   71%
Cholesterol 0mg 0%

Sodium 54mg   2%
Total Carbohydrate 56.1g   20%
Dietary Fiber 20.8g   74%
Total Sugars 21.3g
Protein 18.3g

Roasted Tofu and Bok Choy with Brown Rice

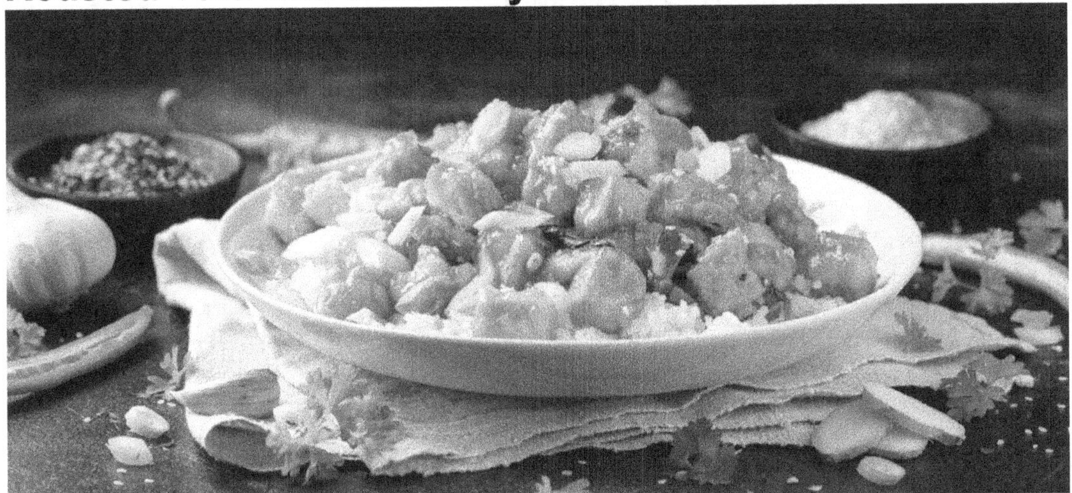

Preparation Time: 15 minutes
Cooking Time: 25-30 minutes
Servings: 4

Ingredients

- 12 ounces block of extra-firm tofu, cut into 2-inch cubes
- 2 red onions, sliced
- 2 cloves garlic crushed and chopped
- 1 teaspoon fresh ginger
- 2 teaspoons sesame oil
- Ground pepper, to taste
- 1/2 tablespoon coconut amino
- 2 teaspoons of agave syrup
- 1 teaspoon of white vinegar
- 1 tablespoon of sesame seeds

Directions

1. Preheat oven to 375 degrees F.
2. In a large bowl add the chopped onions, black pepper, ginger, garlic, coconut amino, and sesame seed.

3. Heat the sesame oil in a cooking pan and cook the bowl ingredients for a few minutes.
4. Add in the Bok Choy and cook for 4 minutes.
5. Set aside for further use.
6. Drain the tofu and cut the tofu block into bite-size pieces.
7. Layer the tofu onto an oil greased baking pan and bake the tofu until golden.
8. Take out the baked tofu from the oven and pour the agave syrup all over.
9. Place the tofu on the serving plate and pour the cooked Bok Choy mixture over.
10. Serve with cooked brown rice with a sprinkle of additional seasoned seeds.

Nutrition Facts

Servings: 4

Amount per serving

Calories   127

% Daily Value*

Total Fat 7g   9%

Saturated Fat 1.2g   6%

Cholesterol 0mg 0%

Sodium 15mg   1%

Total Carbohydrate 10.3g   4%

Dietary Fiber 2.3g   8%

Total Sugars 2.9g

Protein 8g

Tuna with Vegetables and Eggs

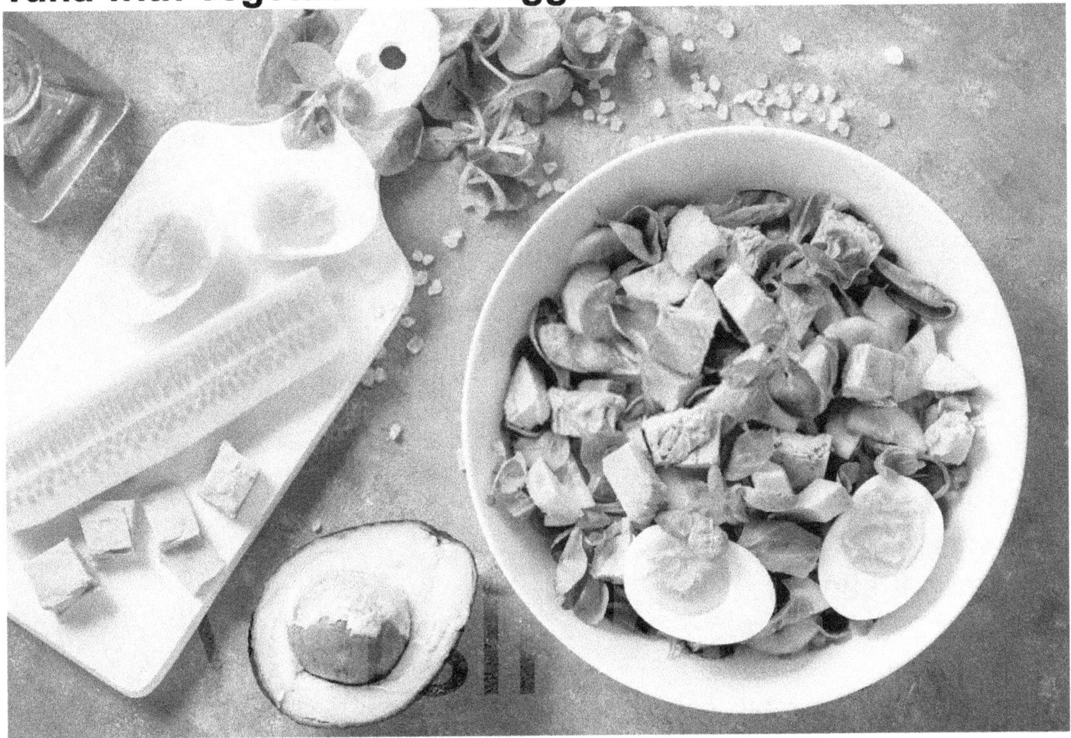

Preparation Time: 15 minutes
Cooking Time: 6 minutes
Servings: 2

Ingredients

- 1 cup of tuna, non-salted and drained
- 4 boiled eggs, diced
- 4tablespoons light mayonnaise
- 1 cup carrots, grated
- Black Pepper to taste

Garnishing

- Few Red chilies
- Few Black Olives, cubed

Directions

1. boil water in a pot enough to hard boil the eggs in it.
2. once done, put the boiled eggs in cold water, then peel the eggs and cut lengthwise.
3. separate the yolks of the eggs and add them to a bowl.
4. now add tuna into the yolks along with, mayonnaise, carrots, and black pepper.
5. Fill the egg whites with this mixture.
6. Garnish at the end with red chilies and olives.
7. Serve and enjoy.

Nutrition Facts

Servings: 4
Amount per serving
Calories   214
% Daily Value*
Total Fat 12.9g   17%
Saturated Fat 2.8g   14%
Cholesterol 181mg   60%
Sodium 207mg   9%
Total Carbohydrate 6.6g   2%
Dietary Fiber 0.7g   2%
Total Sugars 2.6g
Protein 17.7g

Mix Vegetable Curry with Brown Rice

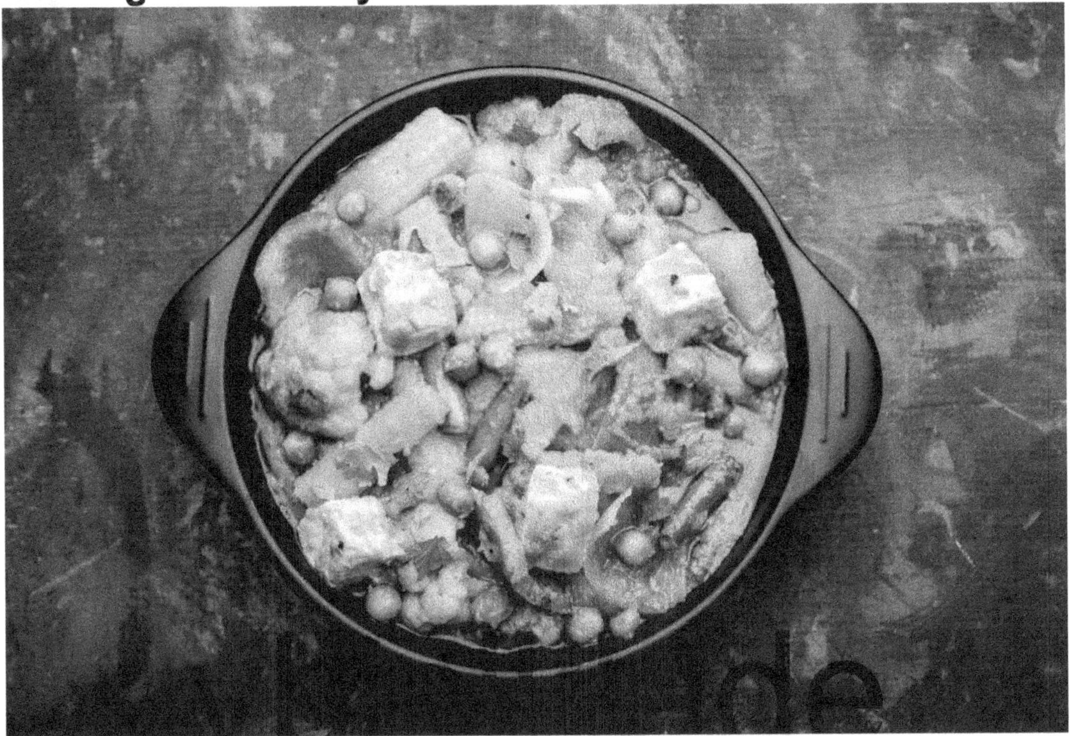

Preparation Time: 20 minutes
Cooking Time: 25 minutes
Servings: 4

Ingredients

- 2 onions, chopped
- ½ teaspoon cumin
- 1 teaspoon red chili flakes
- 1/3 teaspoon cayenne pepper
- 1 cup broccoli,
- 1 cup cabbage
- 1 cup carrot, cubed
- 1 boiled beetroot, washed, peeled
- 4 tablespoons olive oil, for frying

- 1 tablespoon ginger garlic paste
- 2 tablespoons water

Side Servings

- 2 cups of brown rice, steamed

Directions

1. Use a steamer and steam all the vegetables until tender.
2. Next, steam the brown rice as well.
3. Now take a nonstick skillet and heat oil in it, then sauté the onions in it.
4. Next, add ginger and garlic paste
5. Cook for a few seconds.
6. Next, add red chili flakes, cumin, and cayenne pepper.
7. Add some water and add the steamed vegetables.
8. Cover it with the lid and cook for about 4 minutes.
9. Once mixed vegetables are thickened, serve over cooked steamed rice.

Nutrition Facts

Servings: 4
Amount per serving
Calories   555
% Daily Value*
Total Fat 17g   22%
Saturated Fat 2.6g   13%
Cholesterol 0mg 0%
Sodium 113mg   5%
Total Carbohydrate 92.9g   34%
Dietary Fiber 8.2g   29%
Total Sugars 12.6g
Protein 10.6g

Stuffed Tomatoes

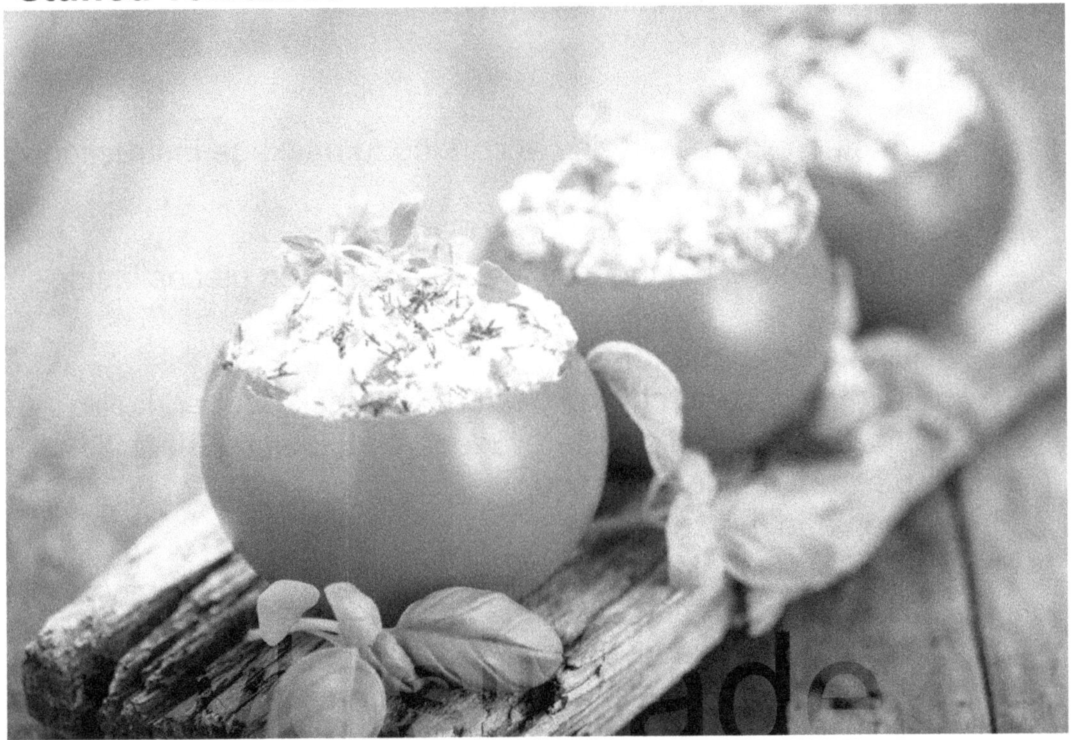

Preparation Time: 25 minutes
Cooking Time: 35 minutes
Servings: 6
Ingredients

- 2 cups uncooked wild rice
- 4 cups vegetable broth, low sodium
- 2 pounds chicken breasts cut in pieces
- 6large red tomatoes
- 4 tablespoons fresh basil
- 4 tablespoons olive oil
- Black pepper, to taste
- 2 tablespoons of lemon juice
- 1/3 teaspoon of red chili powder
- 2 jalape ñ os, chopped

- ¼ teaspoon of Salt-Free Garlic & Herb Seasoning
- ½ teaspoon of Italia seasoning

Directions

1. First, cook the wild rice according to package instructions using vegetable broth.
2. Next, preheat the oven to 400 degrees F.
3. Oil grease a baking tray and cook chicken pieces inside the oven.
4. Center cord the tomatoes.
5. Mix the cooked chicken with basil, black pepper, Italia seasoning, Garlic & Herb Seasoning, jalape ñ o, chili powder, and lemon juice.
6. then add the cooked rice.
7. Mix all the ingredients well
8. then stuff tomatoes with the rice filling.
9. drizzle the olive oil on top.
10. Bake in the oven for 15 minutes.
11. Serve and enjoy.

Nutrition Facts

Servings: 6
Amount per serving
Calories   587
% Daily Value*
Total Fat 22.1g   28%
Saturated Fat 4.8g   24%
Cholesterol 135mg   45%
Sodium 645mg   28%
Total Carbohydrate 41.1g   15%
Dietary Fiber 3.6g   13%
Total Sugars 2.1g
Protein 55g

Lentil and Rice Patties

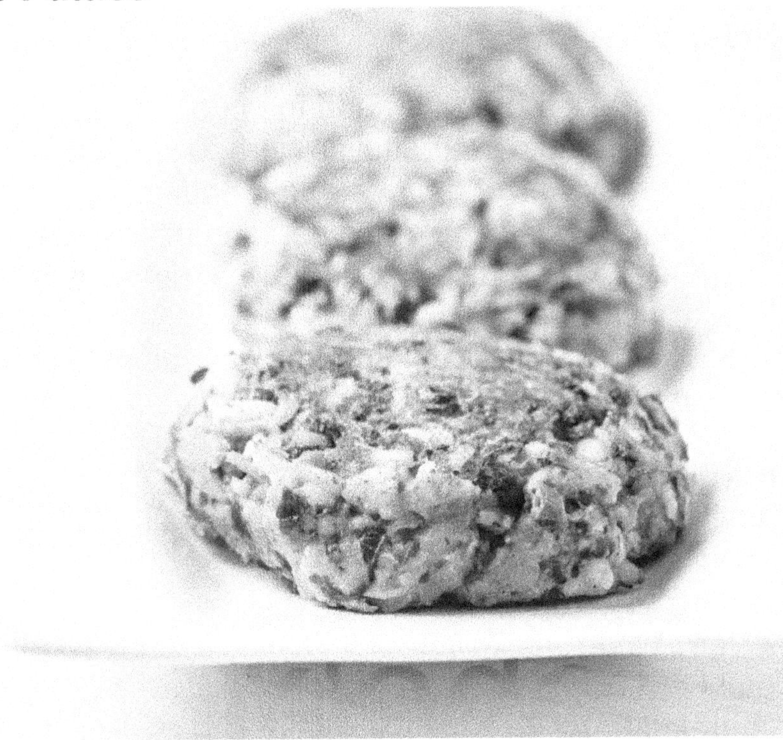

Preparation Time: 20 minutes
Cooking Time: 25 minutes
Servings: 4

Ingredients

- cup brown rice, cooked
- 1 cup brown lentils, cooked
- ½ cup parsley, chopped
- 1 cup carrot, finely grated
- 1/3 cup onion, finely chopped
- 4 clove garlic, minced
- ½ teaspoon ground black pepper
- teaspoons mixed Italian herbs
- tablespoons olive oil

- 1 cup breadcrumbs (use gluten-free)

Directions

1. Take a bowl and add the cooked rice, lentils, parsley, grated carrots, Italian herb, onion, garlic, and black pepper
2. Mix well and make round patties.
3. now start cooking by adding oil to a skillet.
4. Coat each patty with breadcrumbs, and then add it to the skillet.
5. cook the patties from both sides until brown.
6. Serve hot.

Nutrition Facts

Servings: 4

Amount per serving

Calories   449

% Daily Value*

Total Fat 17g   22%

Saturated Fat 2.6g   13%

Cholesterol 0mg 0%

Sodium 349mg   15%

Total Carbohydrate 65.8g   24%

Dietary Fiber 4.9g   17%

Total Sugars 4.5g

Protein 9.5g

Mix Veggies Salad

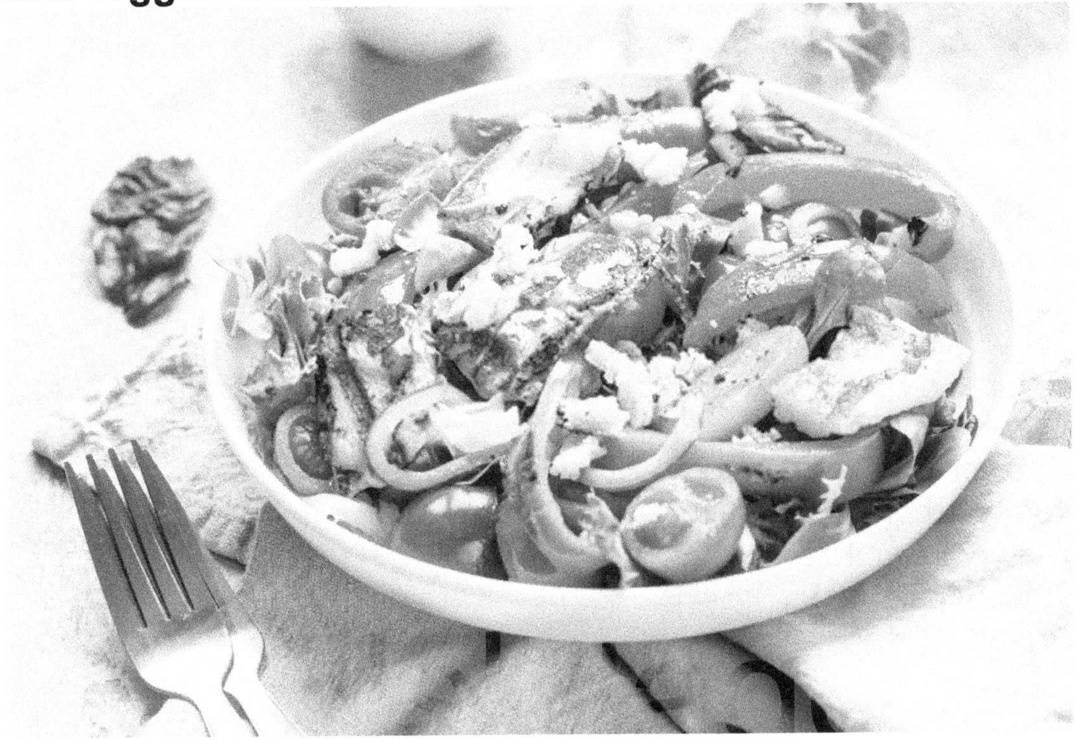

Preparation Time: 5 minutes
Cooking Time: 0 minutes
Servings: 2

Ingredients

- 1 cup cucumber, diced
- 1 cup tomatoes, diced and seeds removed
- 2 tablespoons of fresh Coriander, chopped
- 4 tablespoons lemon juice
- black pepper, to taste
- 2 cups Greek your art
- 1 /3cup green olives, diced

Directions

1   toss all the listed ingredients in a large bowl.
2   stir to combine well
3   once combined, serve fresh.

Nutrition Facts
Servings: 2
Amount per serving
Calories   162
% Daily Value*
Total Fat 3g   4%
Saturated Fat 0.3g   1%
Cholesterol 5mg 2%
Sodium 437mg   19%
Total Carbohydrate 18.1g   7%
Dietary Fiber 1.5g   5%
Total Sugars 12.9g
Protein 13.4g

Marinated Chicken Breasts

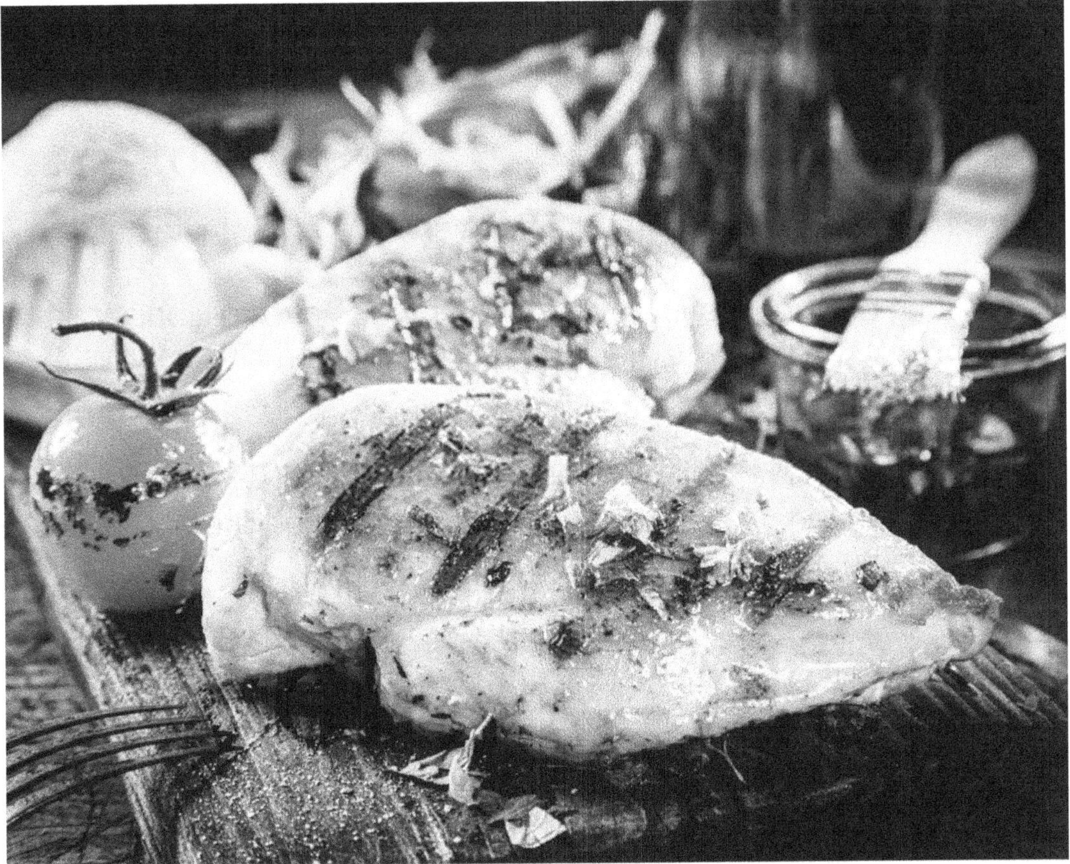

Preparation Time:25 minutes
Cooking Time: 35 minutes
Servings: 4

Ingredients

- tablespoons of olive oil
- 1/4 cup balsamic vinegar
- cloves garlic, minced
- 4 tablespoons of basil, fresh
- 2 teaspoons of red chili powder
- Black pepper, to taste

- 2 pounds of chicken breasts, boneless and skinless
- 1 cup Greek yogurt
- 1 /4 teaspoon of turmeric
- 1 teaspoon of cumin

Directions

1. The first step is to preheat the oven for a few minutes at 400 degrees F.
2. Take a large plastic zip lock bag and add olive oil, balsamic vinegar, basil leaves, garlic, black pepper, red chili powder, cumin, low-fat yogurt, and turmeric.
3. Mix it all well and add the chicken pieces.
4. Mix so the chicken coats well.
5. Then marinate it for 4 hours inside the refrigerators.
6. Take out the chicken just before cooking.
7. Let it sit for 10 minutes.
8. Now put the chicken in an oil greased baking tray and bake for 35 minutes.
9. Once the chicken's internal temperature reaches 165 degrees F, it has done.
10. Serve and enjoy.

Nutrition Facts

Servings: 4

Amount per serving

Calories   793

% Daily Value*

Total Fat 37.3g   48%

Saturated Fat 11.2g   56%

Cholesterol 217mg   72%

Sodium 309mg   13%

Total Carbohydrate 14.3g   5%

Dietary Fiber 0.6g   2%

Total Sugars 12.3g
Protein 96.4g

Rigatoni Noodles with Broccoli

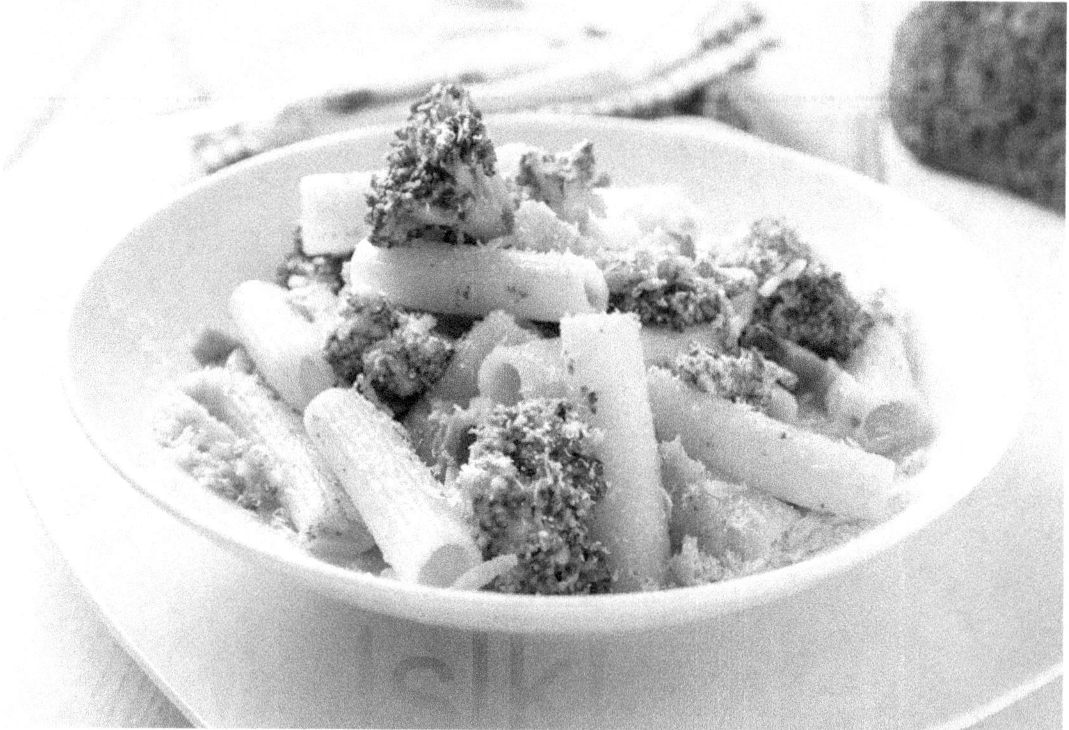

Preparation Time: 20 minutes
Cooking Time: 25 minutes
Servings: 4

Ingredients

- ½ pound rigatoni noodles, whole grain
- ½ cup broccoli florets
- 6 tablespoons of Parmesan cheese
- 2 teaspoons olive oil
- 2 teaspoons garlic, minced
- Black pepper, to taste
- 1 teaspoon of balsamic vinegar

Directions

1   First cook the noodles according to package instructions, then drain and set aside for further use.
2   Steam the broccoli and add it to the cooked noodles.
3   Sprinkle cheese on top along with a drizzle of vinegar, olive oil, garlic, and black pepper.
4   Toss and serve.

Nutrition Facts

Servings: 4

Amount per serving

Calories   557

% Daily Value*

Total Fat 7.8g   10%

Saturated Fat 2.3g   12%

Cholesterol 10mg   3%

Sodium 134mg   6%

Total Carbohydrate 103.8g   38%

Dietary Fiber 5.2g   19%

Total Sugars 2.6g

Protein 19.5g

Lunch Time Mango Salad with Vegetables

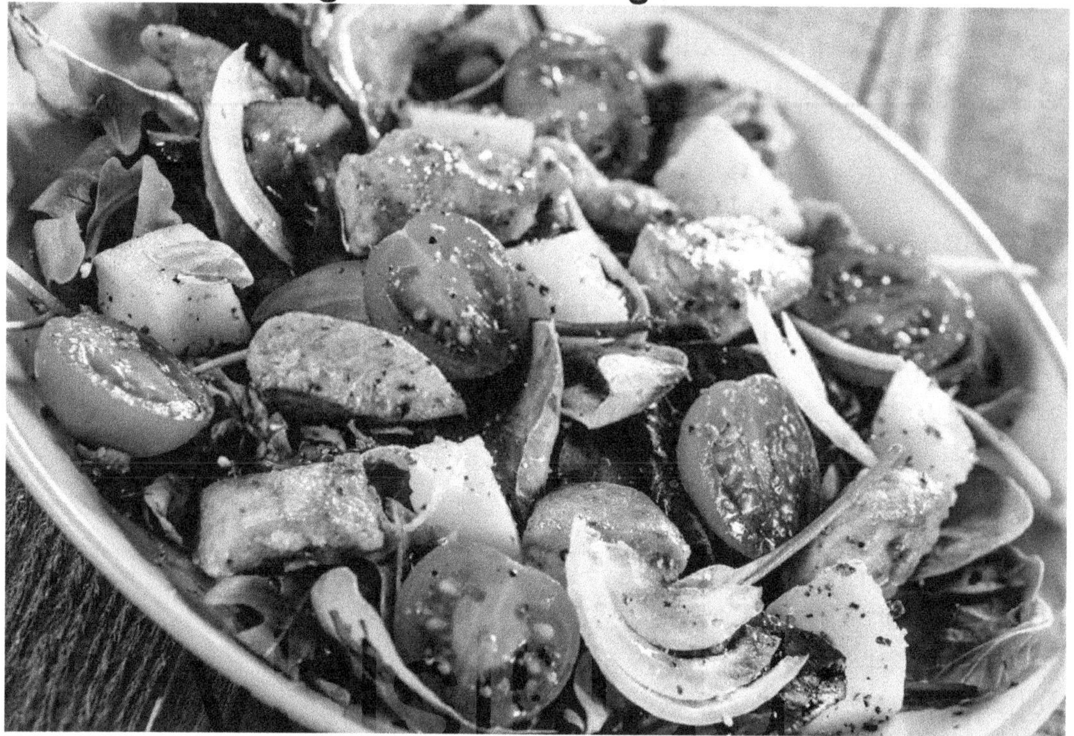

Preparation Time: 6 minutes
Cooking Time: 0 minutes
Servings: 2

Ingredients

- 1/3 cup red onions, sliced
- 1 cup baby spinach
- 2 cups mangoes, peeled and cubed
- 2 tablespoons orange juice
- ¼ teaspoon black pepper
- tablespoons extra virgin olive oil

Directions

1   Take a large bowl and toss together red onions, baby spinach, and mangoes.
2   In a small bowl, mix black pepper, olive oil, and orange juice.
3   Drizzle it over salad and toss.
4   Serve immediately.

Nutrition Facts

Servings: 2

Amount per serving

Calories   298

% Daily Value*

Total Fat 21.8g   28%

Saturated Fat 3.2g   16%

Cholesterol 0mg 0%

Sodium 15mg   1%

Total Carbohydrate 28.8g   10%

Dietary Fiber 3.5g   12%

Total Sugars 24.7g

Protein 2.1g

10 Drink/ Smoothies

Coconut and Avocado Smoothie

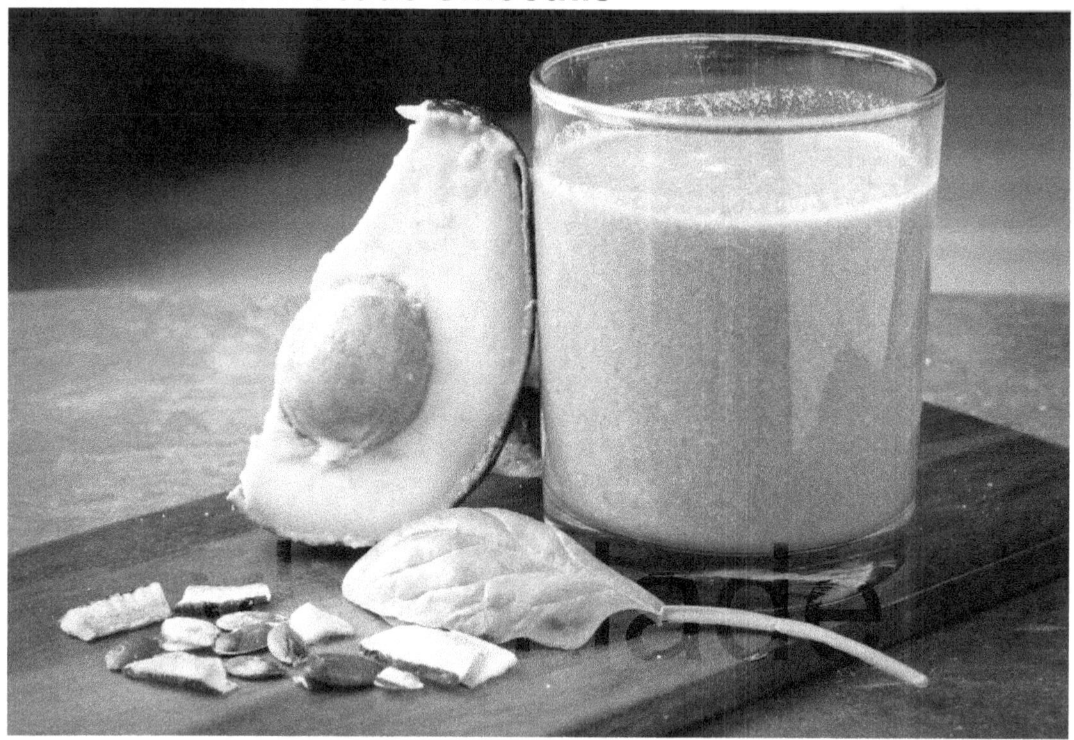

Preparation Time: minutes
Cooking Time: 0 minutes
Servings: 4

Ingredients

- 2 avocados, fresh and pitted
- 2tablespoons of coconut oil
- 2 cups coconut milk
- ½ cup baby spinach
- 1 green apple, peeled

Directions

1   Add all the listed ingredients in a high-speed blender.
2   Pulse all the listed ingredients into a smoothie.
3   Pour into ice-filled tall serving glasses.
4   Serve and enjoy.

Nutrition Facts

Servings: 4
Amount per serving
Calories   570
% Daily Value*
Total Fat 55.1g   71%
Saturated Fat 35.4g   177%
Cholesterol 0mg 0%
Sodium 27mg   1%
Total Carbohydrate 23.1g   8%
Dietary Fiber 10.8g   39%
Total Sugars 10.3g
Protein 4.9g

Energetic Cherry Smoothie

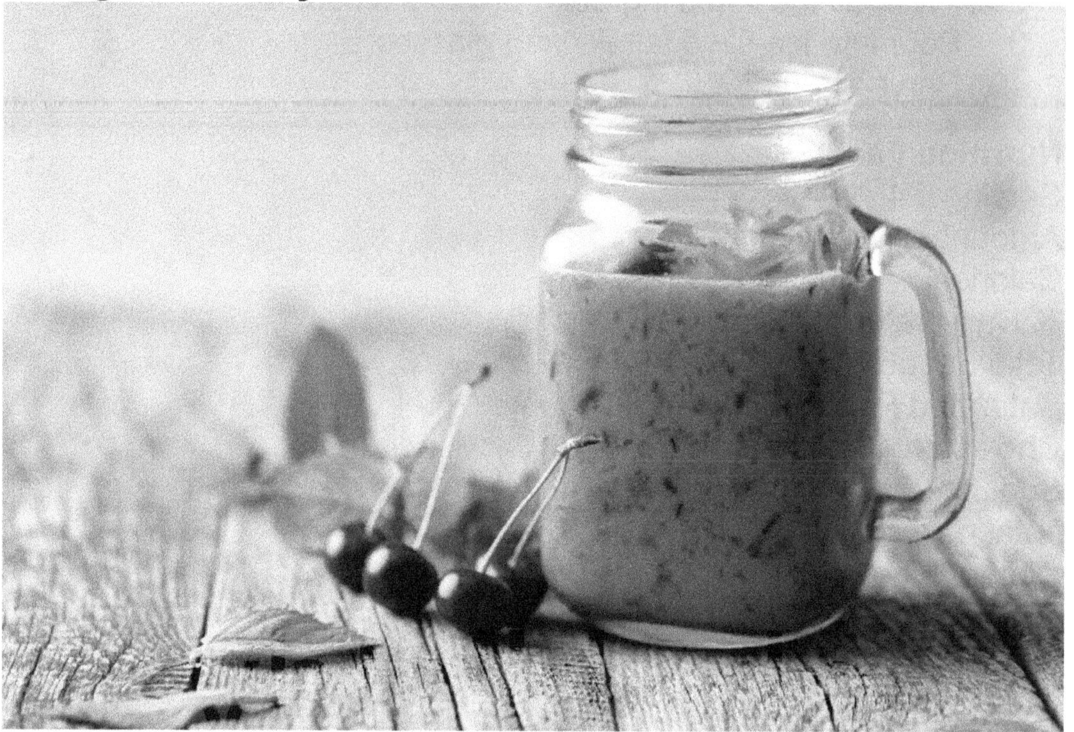

Preparation Time: 6 minutes
Cooking Time: 0 minutes
Servings: 4
Ingredients

- ½ cup Greek yogurt, plain
- 1 cup cherries, stems removed
- 1 tablespoon of Chia seeds
- ½ cup almond milk
- ½ cup spinach
- ½ cup pineapple

Directions

1   The first step is to wash the cherries and then remove the
     pits.
2   Take a blender and add Greek yogurt, cherries, chia seed,
     almond milk, spinach, and pineapple
3   Pulse all the listed ingredients until smooth.
4   Pour it into ice-filled tall serving glasses.
5   Serve and enjoy.

Nutrition Facts
Servings: 4
Amount per serving
Calories   492
% Daily Value*
Total Fat 18.2g   23%
Saturated Fat 9.5g   48%
Cholesterol 8mg 3%
Sodium 123mg   5%
Total Carbohydrate 62.9g   23%
Dietary Fiber 1g 4%
Total Sugars 9.1g
Protein 20.4g

Three Blueberry Smoothies

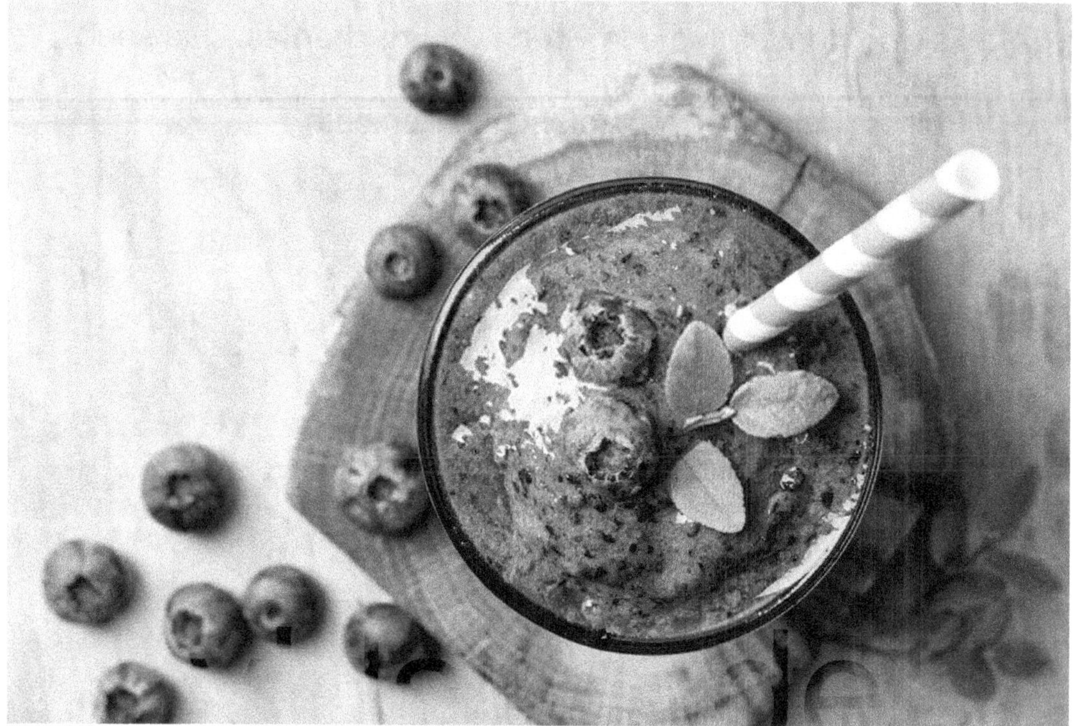

Preparation Time: 12 minutes
Cooking Time: 0 minutes
Servings: 2

Ingredients

- 1 cup blueberries
- 1 cup raspberries
- cup strawberries
- 1 .5 cups coconut milk
- 1 apple, cored and diced
- Ice cubes for chilling

Directions

1   Put all the listed ingredients in a blender.

2   Blend for 1 minute or until smooth.
3   Pour into tall serving glasses.
4   Enjoy chilled.
5

Nutrition Facts

Servings: 2

Amount per serving

Calories   293

% Daily Value*

Total Fat 15.4g   20%

Saturated Fat 12.7g   63%

Cholesterol 0mg 0%

Sodium 12mg   1%

Total Carbohydrate 42.1g   15%

Dietary Fiber 11.2g   40%

Total Sugars 27.1g

Protein 3.4g

Orange and Flax Seed Smoothie

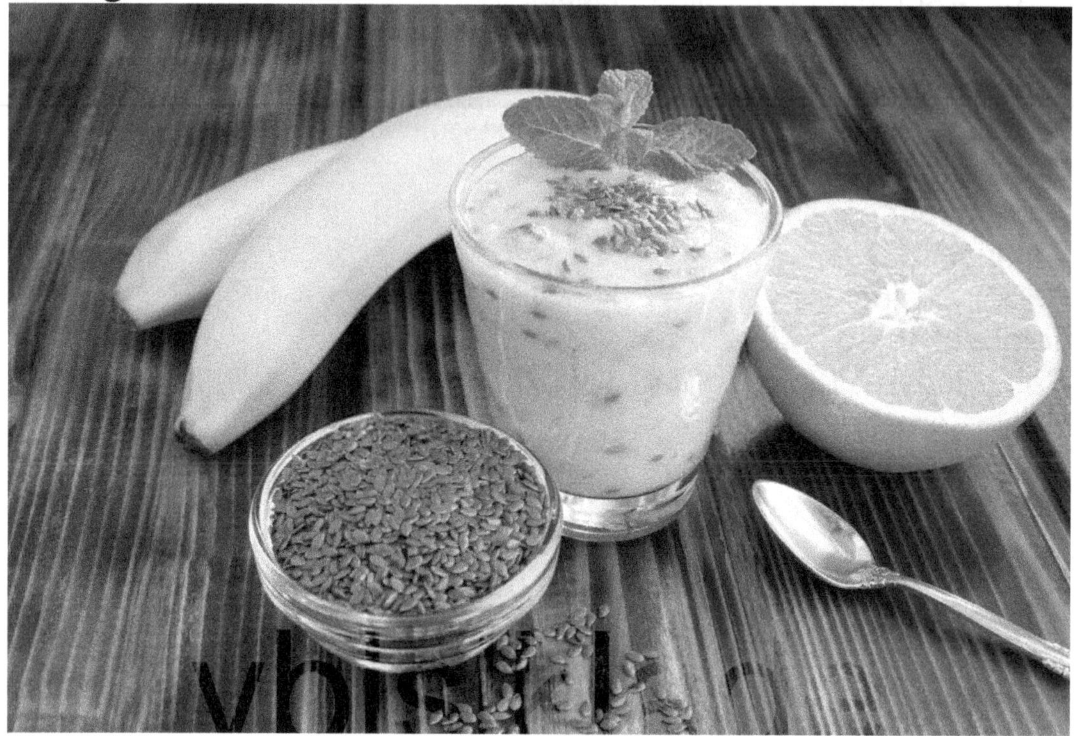

Preparation Time: 12 minutes
Cooking Time:0 minutes
Servings: 2

Ingredients

- 1 cup fresh peaches, sliced and pitted
- 2 cups orange juice, fresh
- 2 tablespoons ground flax seeds
- 2 red apples, seedless and skinless
- 1 cup ice cubes

Directions

1   Put all the listed ingredients in a high-speed blender.
2   Pulse it until smooth.

3   Pour into tall serving glasses.

4   Serve and enjoy.

Nutrition Facts

Servings: 2

Amount per serving

Calories   295

% Daily Value*

Total Fat 3.3g   4%

Saturated Fat 0.4g   2%

Cholesterol 0mg 0%

Sodium 10mg   0%

Total Carbohydrate 65.6g   24%

Dietary Fiber 9g 32%

Total Sugars 51.1g

Protein 4.3g

Watermelon And Peach Smoothie

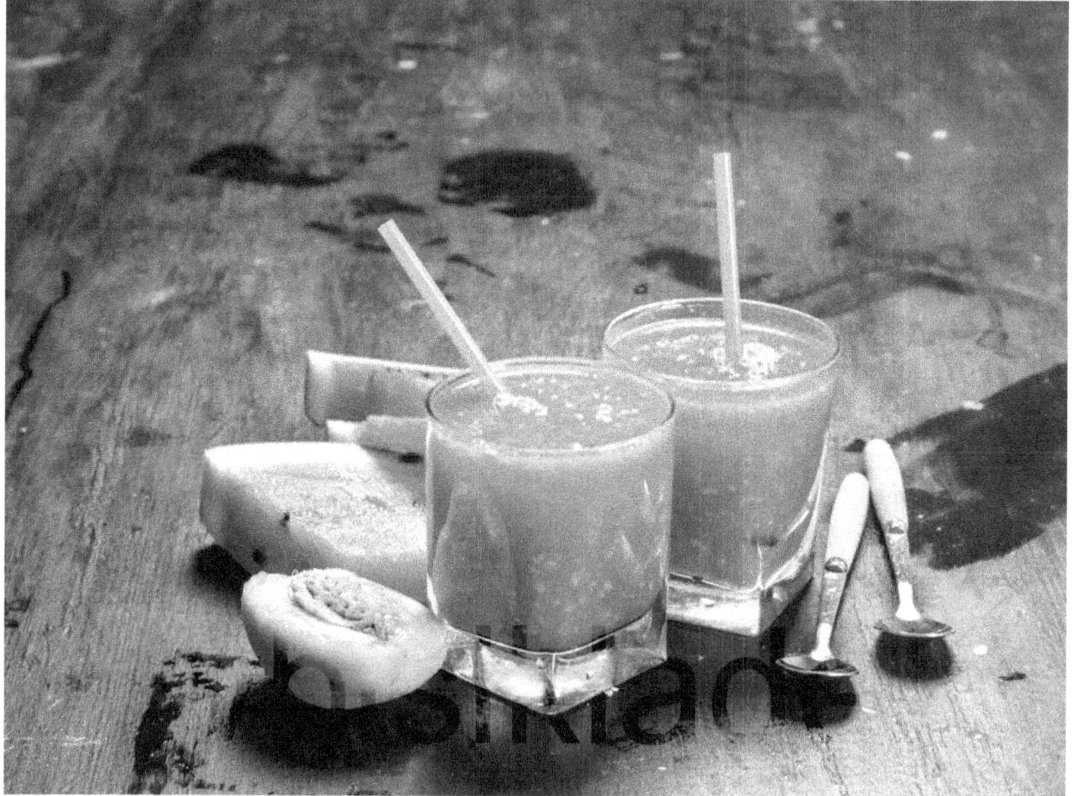

Preparation Time:6 minutes
Cooking Time: 0minutes
Servings: 2

Ingredients

- 2 cups watermelon, cubed and seedless
- 2 peaches, seedless and peeled
- 1 cup organic strawberries
- ½ cup coconut water

Directions

1   Put all the listed ingredients in a blender.

2	Blend for 1 minute or until smooth.
3	Serve chilled.
4	Enjoy.

Nutrition Facts

Servings: 2

Amount per serving

Calories   239

% Daily Value*

Total Fat 12.9g   17%

Saturated Fat 10.8g   54%

Cholesterol 0mg 0%

Sodium 10mg   0%

Total Carbohydrate 32.5g   12%

Dietary Fiber 4.3g   16%

Total Sugars 26.9g

Protein 3.9g

Veggies Smoothie

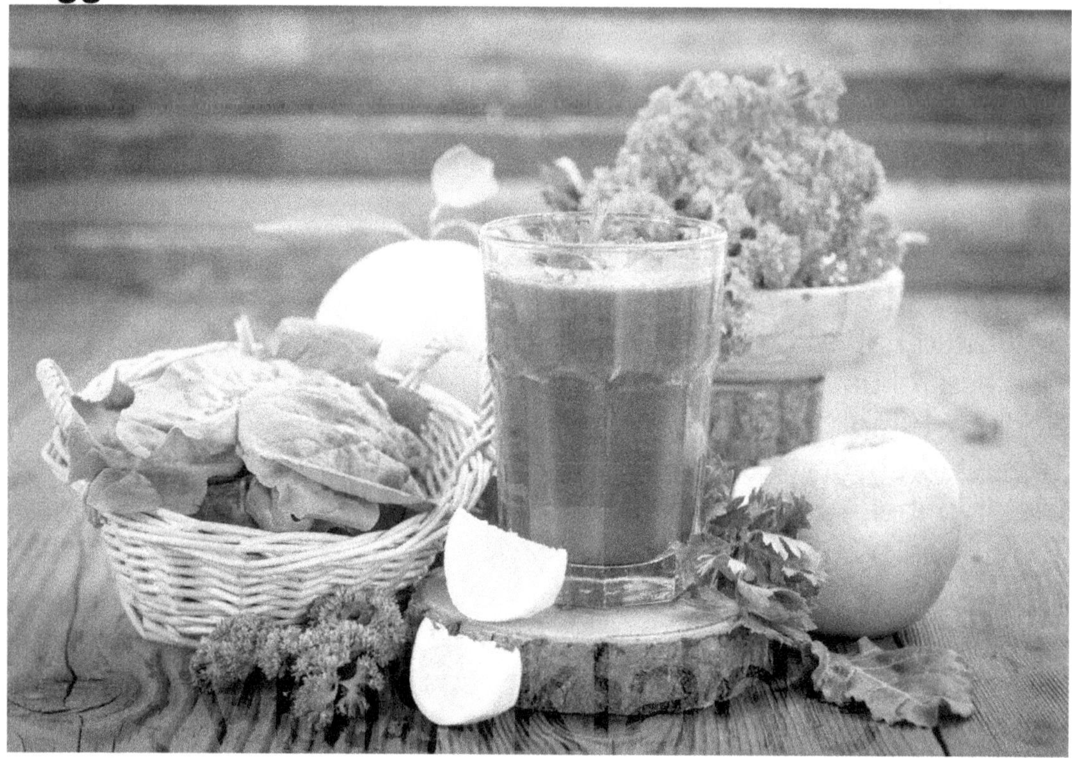

Preparation Time: 6 minutes
Cooking Time: 0 minutes
Servings: 2

Ingredients

- 2 cups kale, washed
- 2 oranges, peeled and seedless
- 1 cup of ice cubes
- 1 cup spinach
- 1 banana, peeled

Directions
1   Put all the listed ingredients in a blender.
2   Blend for 1 minute or until smooth.

3   Serve chilled.
4   Enjoy.

Nutrition Facts

Servings: 2

Amount per serving

Calories   175

% Daily Value*

Total Fat 0.5g   1%

Saturated Fat 0.1g   1%

Cholesterol 0mg 0%

Sodium 45mg   2%

Total Carbohydrate 42.6g   16%

Dietary Fiber 7.3g   26%

Total Sugars 24.5g

Protein 4.8g

Detox Smoothie

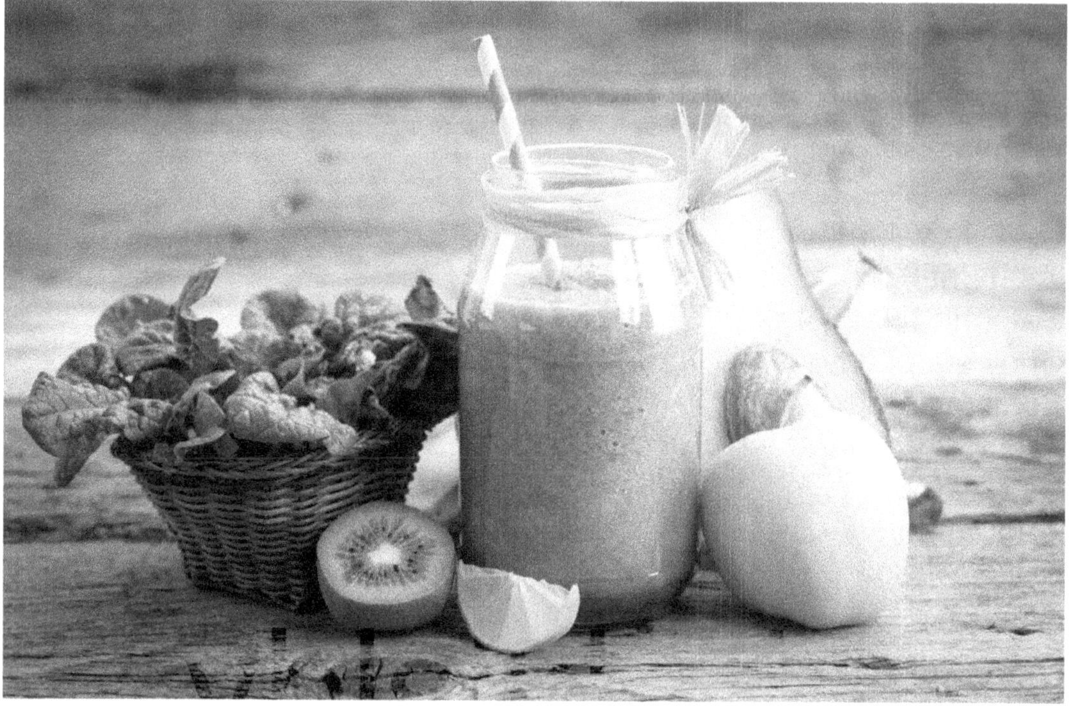

Preparation Time: 7 minutes
Cooking Time: 0 minutes
Servings: 2

Ingredients

- 2 green apples, washed
- 1 cup grapes, washed
- kiwis, washed and peeled
- 1 cup of ice- cubes
- 1 cup coconut water

Directions

1 Take a high-speed blender and add apple grapes, kiwi, kale, and coconut water.

2   Pulse it for 40 seconds.
3   Pour it into glasses
4   Serve and enjoy.

Nutrition Facts
Servings: 2
Amount per serving
Calories   311
% Daily Value*
Total Fat 1.8g   2%
Saturated Fat 0.1g   1%
Cholesterol 0mg 0%
Sodium 47mg   2%
Total Carbohydrate 78.6g   29%
Dietary Fiber 12.7g   45%
Total Sugars 57.2g
Protein 3.5g

Oat Cocoa Smoothie

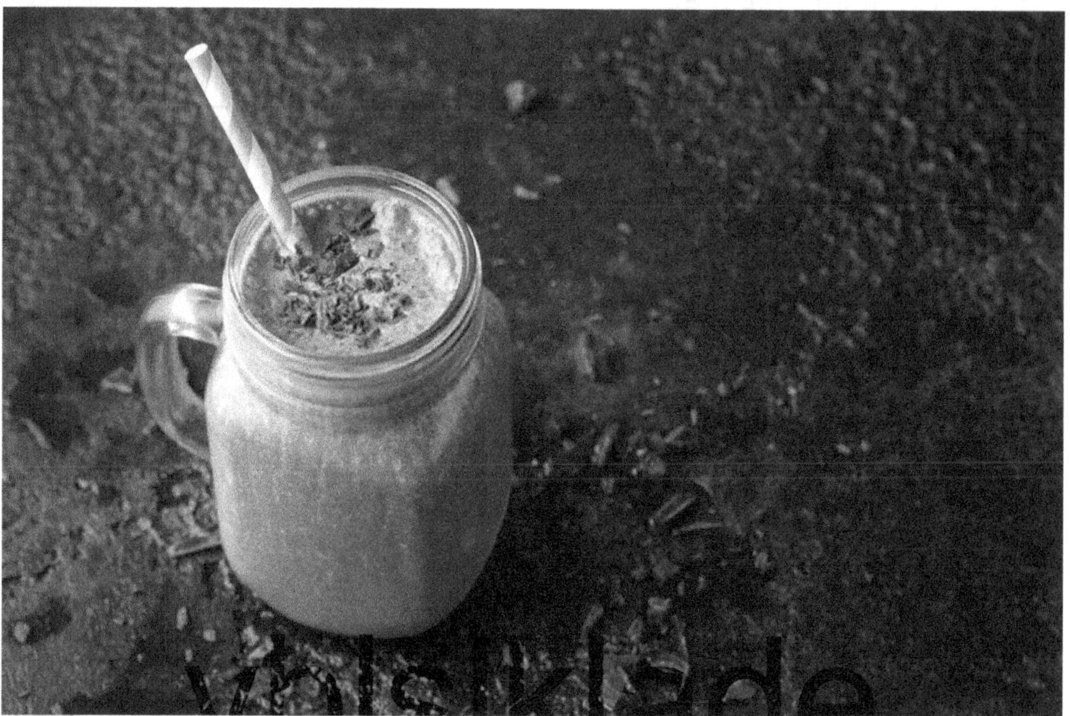

Preparation Time: 6 minutes
Cooking Time: 0 minutes
Servings: 2

Ingredients

- 3/4 cup skim milk
- ½ teaspoon vanilla extract
- 1 cup plain low-fat yogurt
- 1/3 cup quick-cook oats
- 2 teaspoons ground flaxseed
- 2 tablespoons unsweetened cocoa powder
- Pinch of cinnamon
- 1 small banana, frozen and peeled

Directions

1. Put all ingredients in a high-speed blender.
2. Blend on medium for 30 seconds, then serve chilled.

Nutrition Facts

Servings: 2
Amount per serving
Calories   222
% Daily Value*
Total Fat 3.7g   5%
Saturated Fat 2g 10%
Cholesterol 9mg 3%
Sodium 138mg   6%
Total Carbohydrate 33.2g   12%
Dietary Fiber 4.5g   16%
Total Sugars 19.7g
Protein 13g

Go Green Smoothies

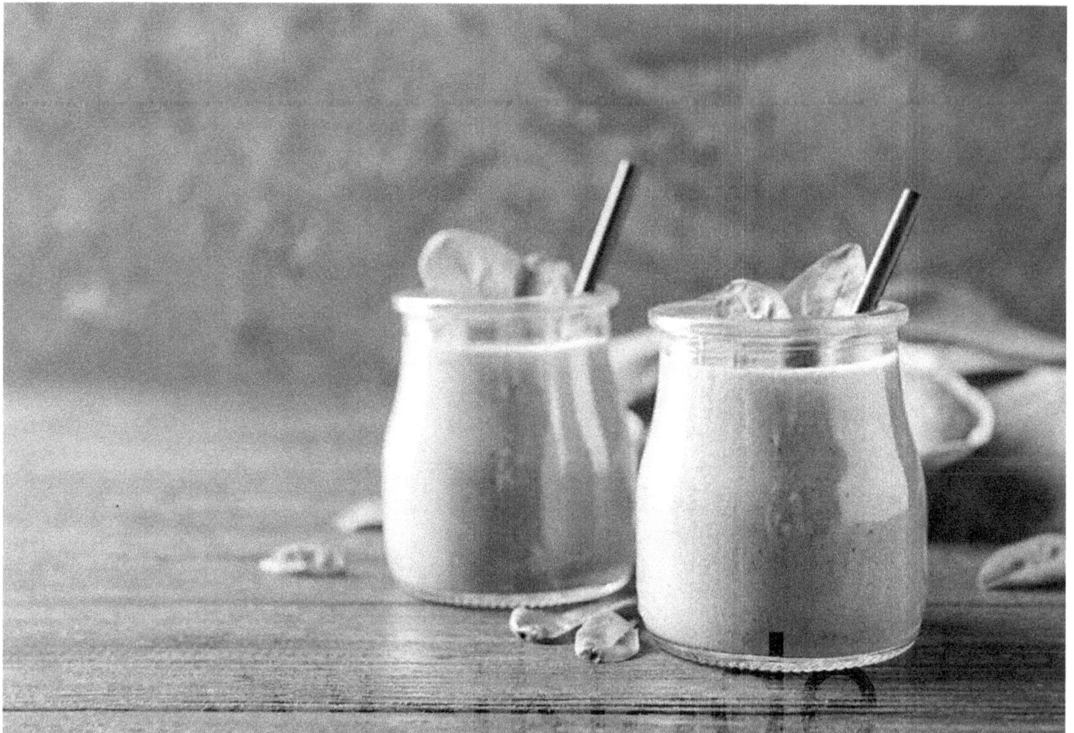

Preparation Time: 8 minutes
Cooking Time: 0 minutes
Servings: 2

Ingredients

- ½ cup broccoli washed
- ½ cucumber washed
- 1 bunch of parsley, washed
- 1 bunch of baby spinach, washed
- apples
- 2 cups pineapple
- Ice cubes, for chilling

Directions

1. Put all the listed ingredients in a high-speed blender.
2. Blend for a few minutes.
3. Pour it into serving glasses and enjoy.

Nutrition Facts
Servings: 2
Amount per serving
Calories   353
% Daily Value*
Total Fat 1.7g   2%
Saturated Fat 0.1g   1%
Cholesterol 0mg 0%
Sodium 140mg   6%
Total Carbohydrate 89.4g   33%
Dietary Fiber 16.8g   60%
Total Sugars 63.4g
Protein 7g

Morning Glory

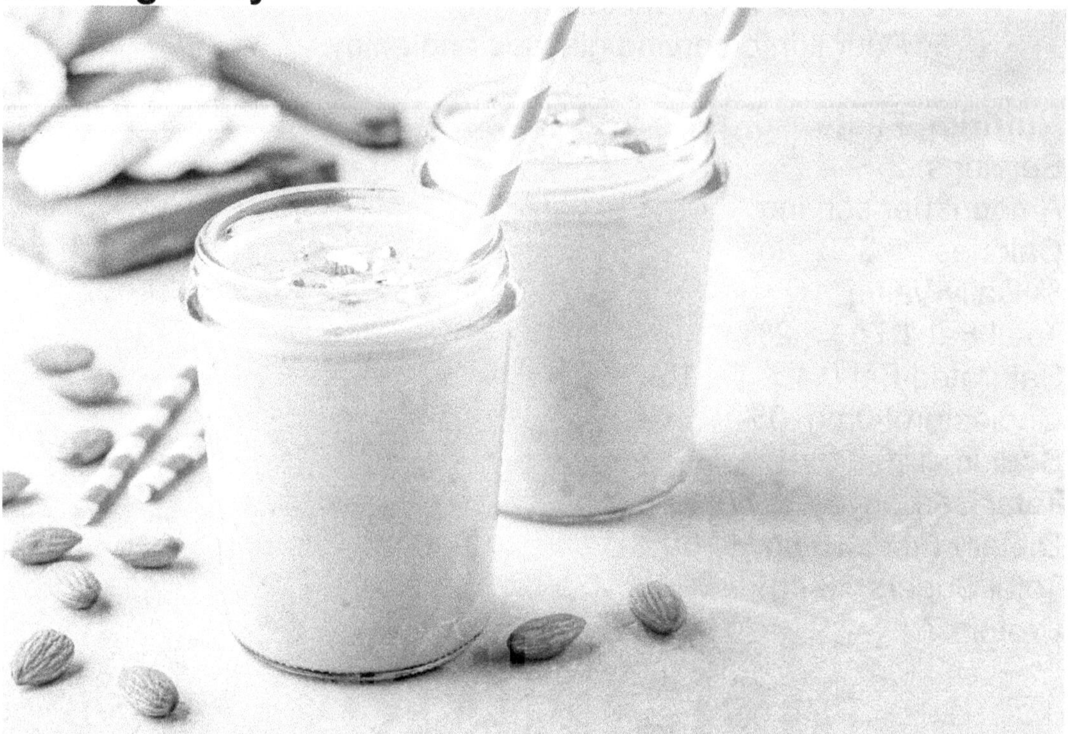

Preparation Time: 7 minutes
Cooking Time: 0 minutes
Servings: 2

Ingredients

- 1 cup almond milk
- 1/3 cup apple juice
- 4 tablespoons walnuts
- 4 tablespoons unsweetened coconut flakes
- 4 frozen bananas
- ½ teaspoon ground cinnamon
- ½ teaspoon pure vanilla extract
- ½ teaspoon stevia
- 1 cup ice cubes

Directions

1. Put the almond milk, apple juice, walnuts, coconut flakes, banana, cinnamon, vanilla extract, stevia, and ice cubes.
2. Blend for a few minutes.
3. Pour it into serving glasses and enjoy.

Nutrition Facts

Servings: 2
Amount per serving
Calories   614
% Daily Value*
Total Fat 39.1g   50%
Saturated Fat 26.6g   133%
Cholesterol 0mg 0%
Sodium 30mg   1%
Total Carbohydrate 68.2g   25%
Dietary Fiber 10.4g   37%
Total Sugars 37.8g
Protein 9.1g

10 Appetizer Recipes

Basil Pesto Stuffed Mushrooms

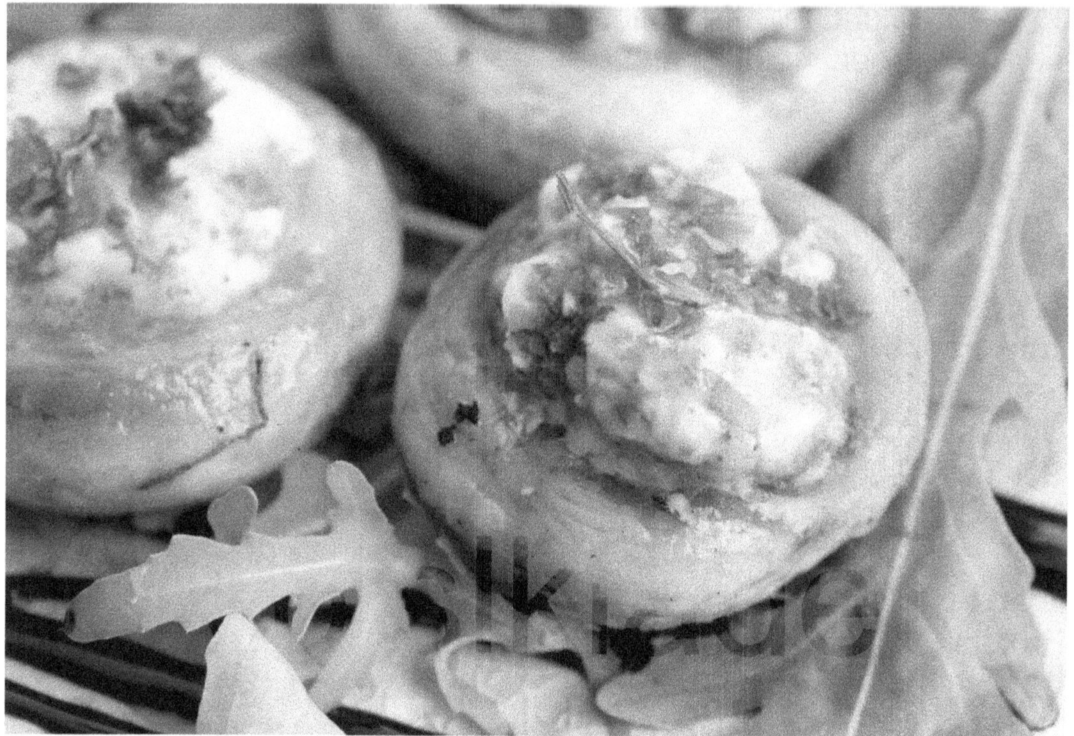

Preparation Time: 15 minutes
Cooking Time:12 minutes
Servings: 3

Ingredients

- 18 cremini mushrooms, stems removed

Topping:

- 1/3 cup melted butter
- 2 cups Panko breadcrumbs
- 4 tablespoons chopped fresh parsley

- Filling:
- 2 cups fresh basil leaves
- 1/2 cup fresh Parmesan cheese
- 3 tablespoons pumpkin seeds
- 2 tablespoons olive oil
- 2 tablespoons fresh garlic
- 2 teaspoons lemon juice

Directions

1. preheat the oven to 375 degrees F.
2. place the mushrooms on the baking sheet upside down.
3. Take a small bowl and mix Panko, butter, and parsley.
4. next put the basil, cheese, oil, pumpkin seeds, garlic, and lemon juice in a food processor and pulse until mixed.
5. next, stuff the cavity of the mushroom with the pesto filling.
6. Sprinkle some Panko topping on top of each mushroom afterward.
7. Bake for 10 to 12 minutes, then serve

Nutrition Facts

Servings: 3
Amount per serving
Calories   1355
% Daily Value*
Total Fat 109.6g 141%
Saturated Fat 64.7g   323%
Cholesterol 237mg   79%
Sodium 1151mg 50%
Total Carbohydrate 75.3g   27%
Dietary Fiber 2.6g   9%
Total Sugars 0.4g
Protein 23g

Black Bean and Corn Relish

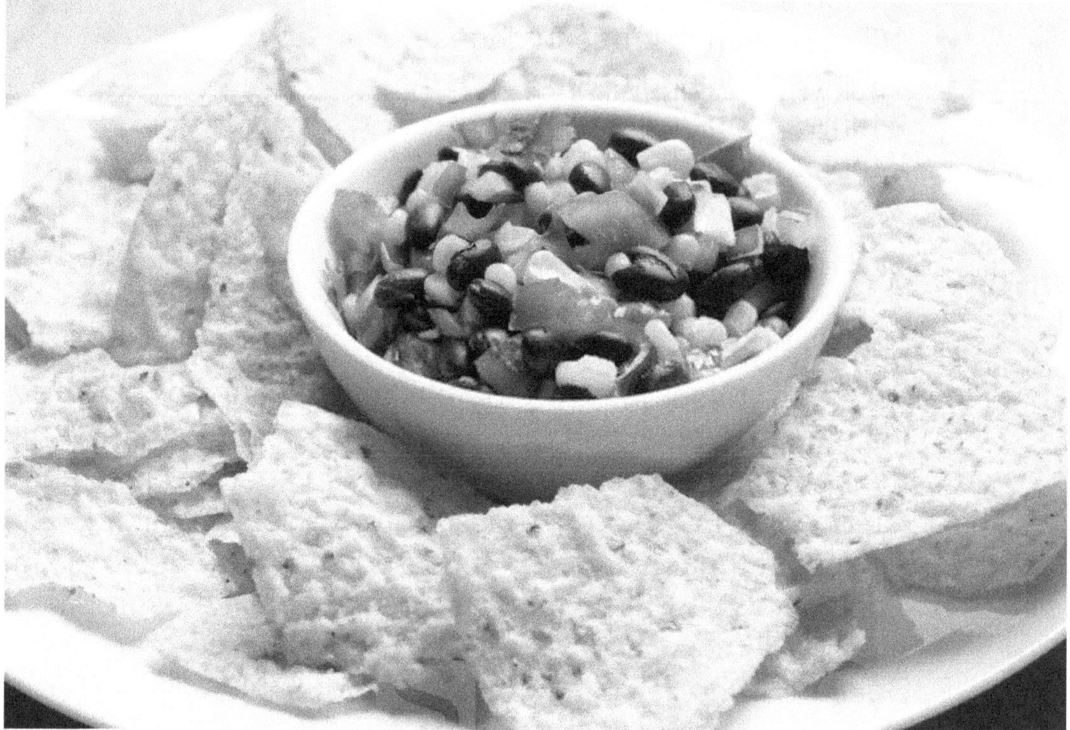

Preparation Time: 15 minutes
Cooking Time: 0 minutes
Servings: 2

Ingredients

- 16 ounces of black beans, cooked
- 1.5 cup frozen corn kernels, thawed
- 4 tomatoes, diced
- 3 garlic cloves, chopped
- 1 medium red onion, diced (about 1/2 cup)
- 1/3 cup chopped parsley
- 1 red bell pepper, seeded and diced (about 1 cup)
- 1 tablespoon of lemon juice

Directions

1. Take a large bowl and add bell pepper, black beans, corn, tomatoes, garlic cloves, parsley, onion, and lemon juice.
2. Mix it very well.
3. Refrigerate for at least 20 minutes
4. Once the flavors blend, serve.

Nutrition Facts

Servings: 2
Amount per serving
Calories   325
% Daily Value*
Total Fat 28.8g   37%
Saturated Fat 25.4g   127%
Cholesterol 0mg 0%
Sodium 24mg   1%
Total Carbohydrate 18.5g   7%
Dietary Fiber 3.8g   14%
Total Sugars 11.7g
Protein 3.1g

Chipotle Spiced Shrimp

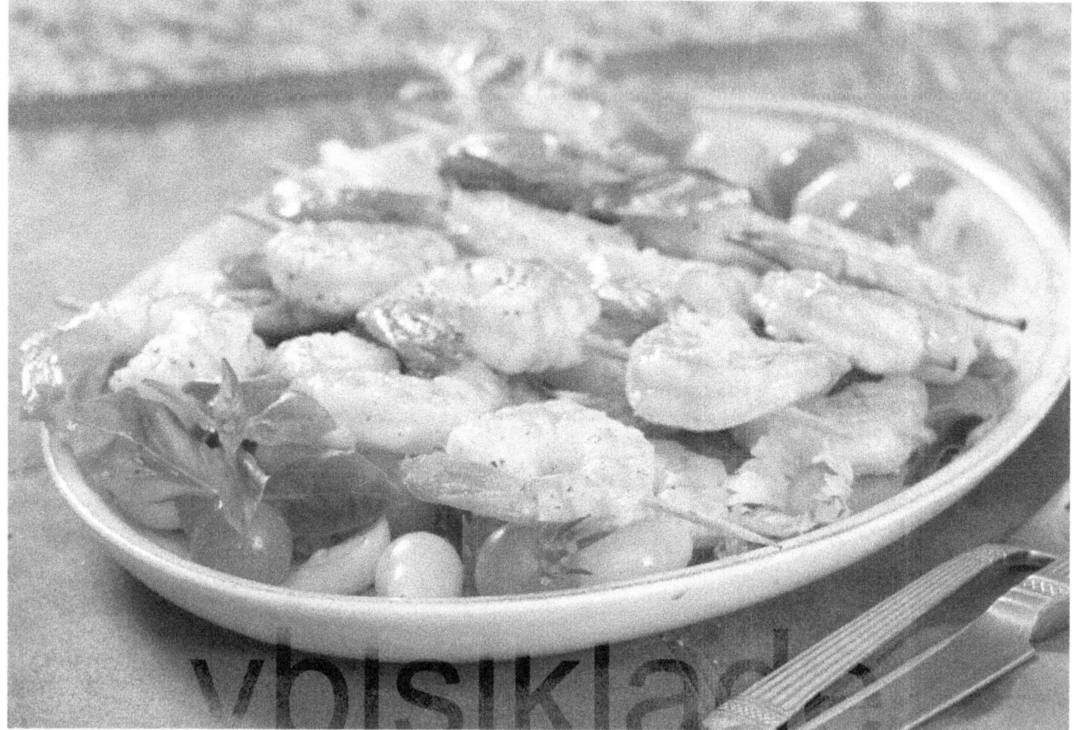

Preparation Time: 15 minutes
Cooking Time: 12 minutes
Servings: 2

Ingredients

- 1-pound uncooked shrimp, peeled and deveined
- 4 tablespoons tomato paste
- 2 teaspoons water
- 1/3 teaspoon extra-virgin olive oil
- 1/3 teaspoon minced garlic
- 1/3 teaspoon chipotle chili powder
- 1/3 teaspoon chopped fresh oregano

Directions

1. rinse and pat dry the shrimp.
2. Take a small bowl and mix the water, tomato paste, oil, garlic, chili powder, and oregano.
3. mix the ingredients well.
4. spread the marinade onto the shrimps and marinate in the refrigerator for 2 hours.
5. Prepare a gas grill or broiler and grease the rack with oil spray.
6. place the shrimp in a grill basket and add it to the grill.
7. Turn the shrimp after 4 minutes.
8. once the shrimp get cooked, serve hot.

Nutrition Facts
Servings: 2
Amount per serving
Calories   304
% Daily Value*
Total Fat 4.8g   6%
Saturated Fat 1.3g   7%
Cholesterol 478mg   159%
Sodium 585mg   25%
Total Carbohydrate 9.8g   4%
Dietary Fiber 1.4g   5%
Total Sugars 3.9g
Protein 53.1g

Coconut Shrimp

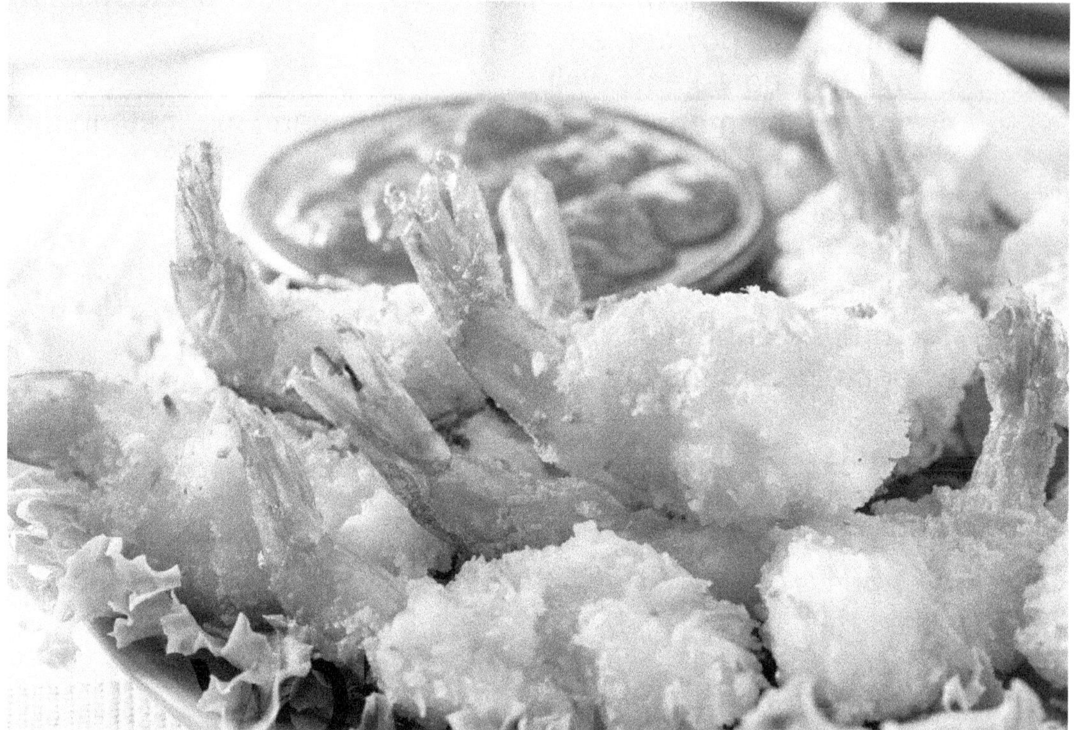

Preparation Time: 15 minutes
Cooking Time: 15 minutes
Servings: 2

Ingredients

- 1/3 cup sweetened coconut
- 1/3 cup Panko breadcrumbs
- 1/2 cup coconut milk
- 10-14 large shrimp, peeled and deveined

Directions

1. Preheat the oven to 375 degrees F.
2. Grease the baking sheet with oil spray.

3. Add the coconut flakes, Panko to a food processor
4. Pulse it to even consistency.
5. put the Panko mixture in a separate bowl.
6. Place the coconut milk in another bowl.
7. Coat each shrimp in the coconut milk and then in the Panko mixture.
8. Add the shrimps to a baking sheet.
9. Lightly coat the top of the shrimp with cooking spray.
10. Bake for about 10 to 15 minutes in preheated oven.
11. Once it is cooked, serve.

Nutrition Facts
Servings: 2
Amount per serving
Calories   230
% Daily Value*
Total Fat 19.3g   25%
Saturated Fat 16.8g   84%
Cholesterol 58mg   19%
Sodium 102mg   4%
Total Carbohydrate 8.3g   3%
Dietary Fiber 2.9g   10%
Total Sugars 2.9g
Protein 8.4g

Crispy Potato Skins

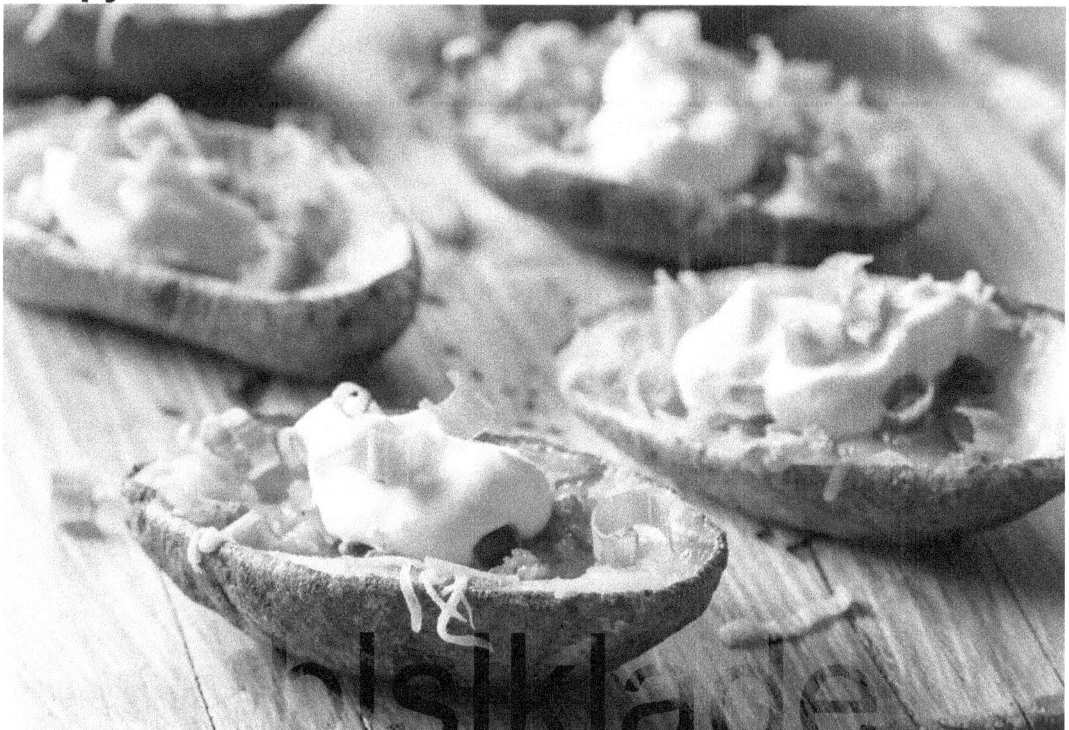

Preparation Time: 15 minutes
Cooking Time: 80 minutes
Servings: 2

Ingredients

- 4 medium russet potatoes
- Butter-flavored cooking spray
- 4 tablespoon minced fresh rosemary
- 1/4 teaspoon black pepper

Directions

1. Preheat the oven to 400 degrees F.

2. wash well the potatoes and then pierce potatoes with a fork.
3. Put the potatoes onto a baking dish and bake in the oven for 60 minutes.
4. take out cooked potatoes and cut the potatoes in half and scoop out the pulp.
5. left about 1/8 inch of the potato flesh attached.
6. Spray the inside of each potato skin with butter-flavored cooking spray.
7. Bake again in the oven for 10 minutes. Serve and enjoy with a sprinkle of rosemary and black pepper.

Nutrition Facts
Servings: 2
Amount per serving
Calories   316
% Daily Value*
Total Fat 1.4g   2%
Saturated Fat 0.6g   3%
Cholesterol 0mg 0%
Sodium 29mg   1%
Total Carbohydrate 71.3g   26%
Dietary Fiber 13.1g   47%
Total Sugars 4.9g
Protein 7.5g

Tomato basil Bruschetta

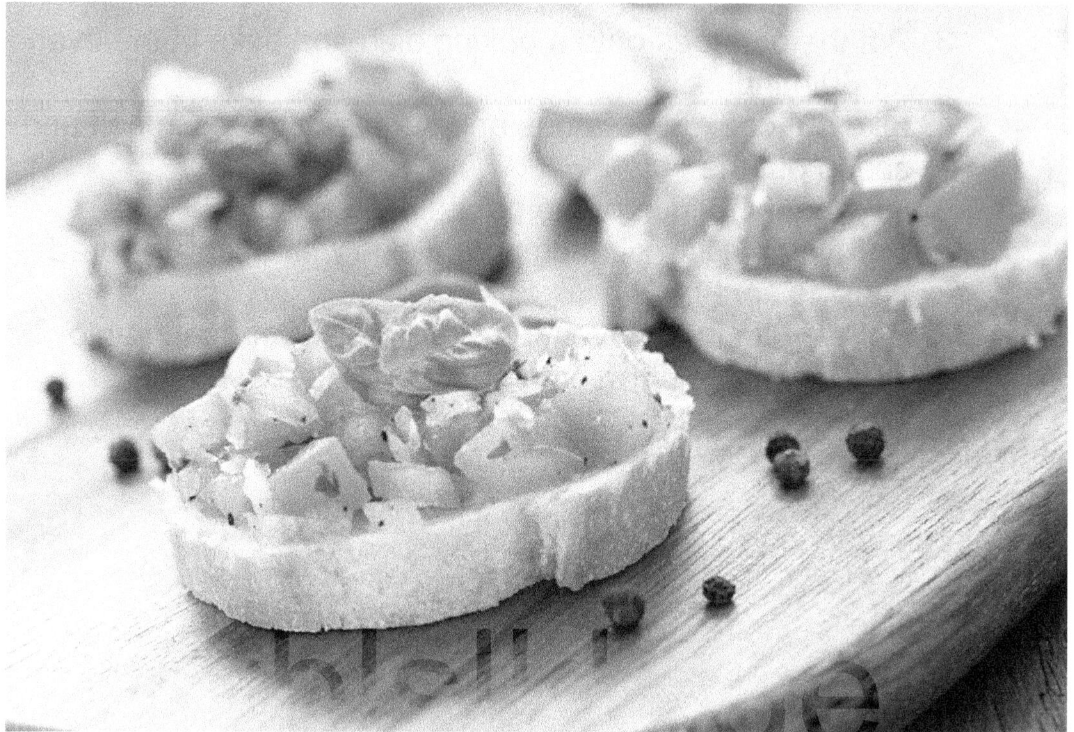

Preparation Time: 15 minutes
Cooking Time: 0 minutes
Servings: 2

Ingredients

- 1 whole-grain baguette, cut into thick diagonal slices
- 4 tablespoons basil, chopped
- 4 tablespoons parsley, chopped
- 4 cloves garlic, minced
- 4 tomatoes, diced
- 1/3 cup diced fennel
- 2 teaspoons olive oil
- 2 teaspoons balsamic vinegar
- ½ teaspoon black pepper

Directions

1. Preheat the oven to 400 degrees F.
2. the first step is to toast the baguette slices until golden.
3. take a bowl and combine well all the other ingredients together.
4. next, spoon the mixture evenly over bread.
5. Serve immediately and enjoy.

Nutrition Facts

Servings: 2
Amount per serving
Calories   664
% Daily Value*
Total Fat 11.3g   15%
Saturated Fat 2.4g   12%
Cholesterol 0mg 0%
Sodium 1106mg 48%
Total Carbohydrate 113.6g   41%
Dietary Fiber 16g   57%
Total Sugars 14.6g
Protein 27.2g

Shrimp With Lime and Dijon Mustard

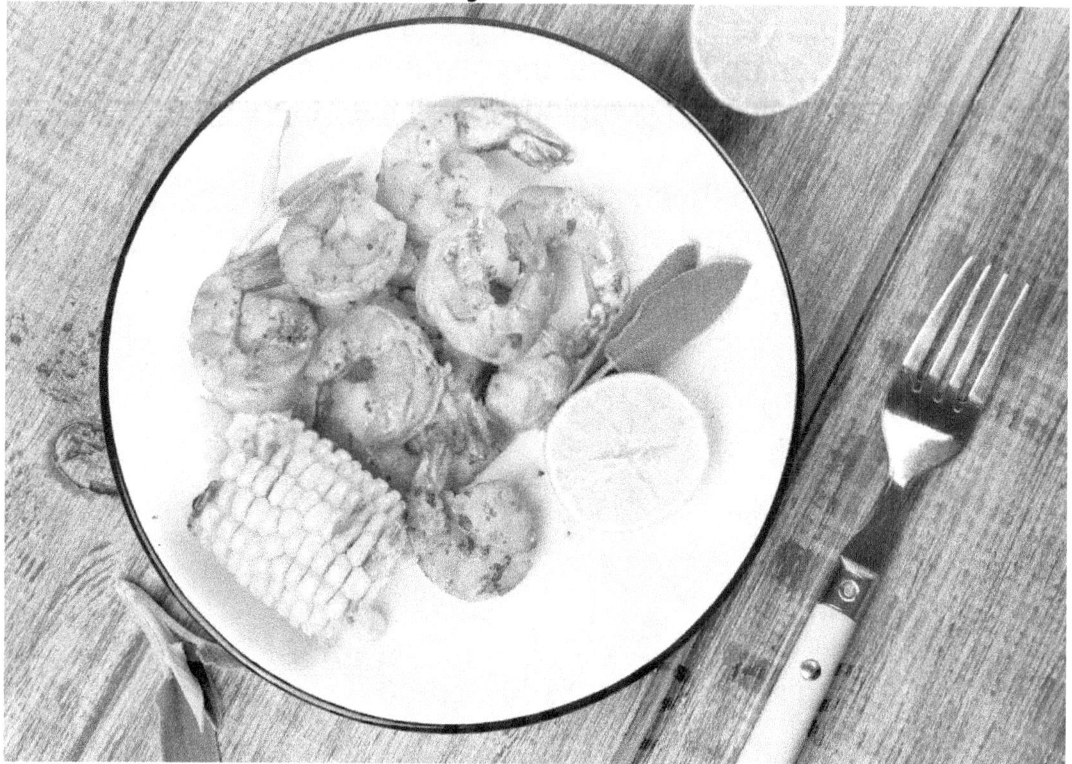

Preparation Time:15 minutes
Cooking Time: 10 minutes
Servings: 2

Ingredients

- 2medium red onion, chopped
- 1 cup fresh lime juice, plus lime zest as garnish
- 4 tablespoons capers
- 2 tablespoon Dijon mustard
- 1 teaspoon hot sauce
- 2 cups water
- 1 cup rice vinegar
- 6 whole cloves

- 2 bay leaf
- 2 pounds uncooked shrimp, peeled and deveined (about 24)

Directions

1. Mix lime juice, onion, mustard, hot sauce, and capers.
2. In a cooking pan or saucepan pour water and add vinegar, bay leaf, and cloves.
3. Bring this mixture to a boil.
4. Then add shrimp and simmer for a few minutes. Then drain and transfer the shrimp to a bowl that contains an onion mixture.
5. discard the bay leaf and cloves.
6. let it refrigerate for a few hours.
7. now to serve it divide it into small bowls and garnish with lime zest

Nutrition Facts

Servings: 2
Amount per serving
Calories   678
% Daily Value*
Total Fat 8.6g   11%
Saturated Fat 2.4g   12%
Cholesterol 955mg   318%
Sodium 1869mg 81%
Total Carbohydrate 18.9g   7%
Dietary Fiber 3.4g   12%
Total Sugars 4.9g
Protein 105.6g

Roasted Butternut Squash Fries

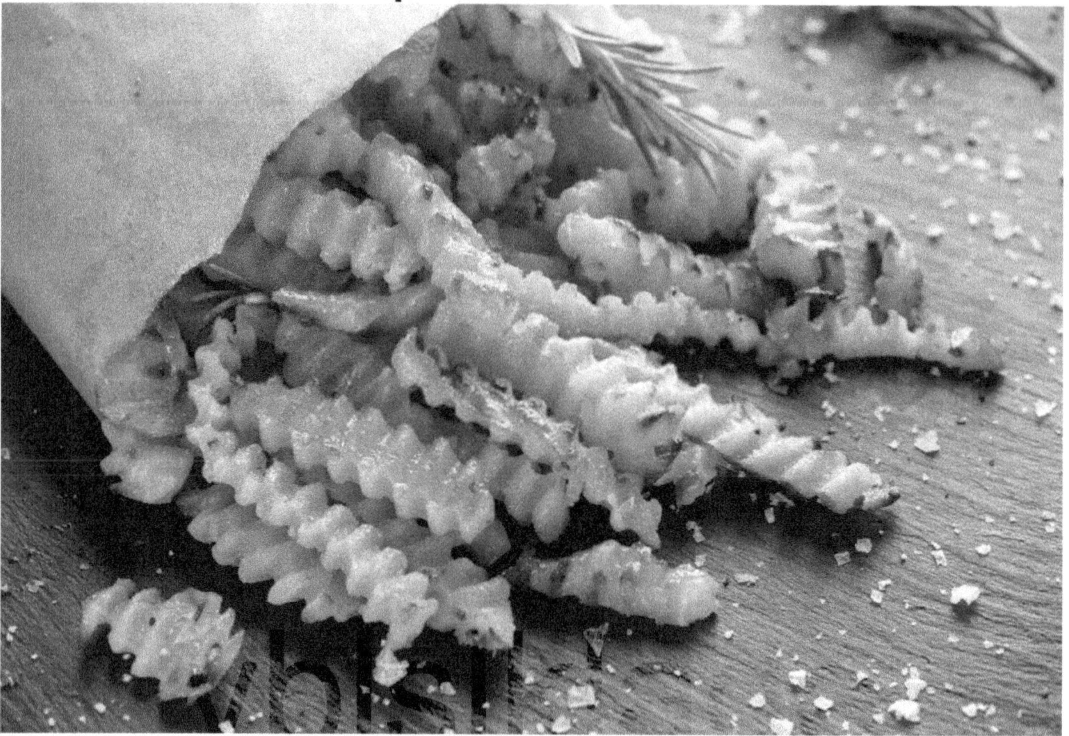

Preparation Time: 15 minutes
Cooking Time: 12 minutes
Servings: 2

Ingredients

- 2 medium butternut squash
- 2 tablespoons olive oil
- 2 tablespoons chopped fresh thyme
- 2 tablespoons chopped fresh rosemary

Directions

1. Preheat the oven to 400 degrees F.
2. Grease a baking sheet with oil spray.

3. Peel the butternut squash and cut it sticks.
4. Combine it with thyme, oil, and rosemary.
5. Toss to coat it well.
6. Layer it onto the baking tray.
7. Cook in the oven for 12 minutes, or until golden brown
8. Serve it hot.

Nutrition Facts
Servings: 2
Amount per serving
Calories   201
% Daily Value*
Total Fat 14.8g   19%
Saturated Fat 2.3g   12%
Cholesterol 0mg 0%
Sodium 9mg   0%
Total Carbohydrate 20.2g   7%
Dietary Fiber 5.2g   19%
Total Sugars 3.1g
Protein 1.8g

Pickled Asparagus

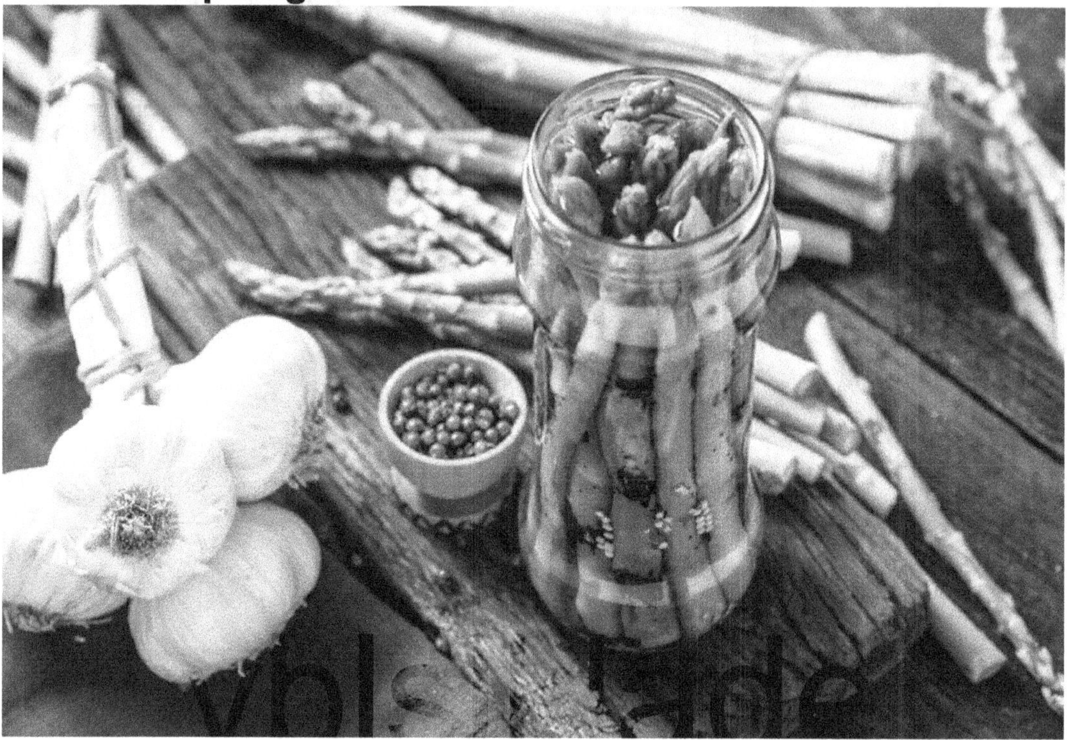

Preparation Time: 15 minutes
Cooking Time:0 minutes
Servings: 2

Ingredients

- 3 cups asparagus, trimmed
- 1/2 cup pearl onions
- 1/4 cup white wine vinegar
- 1/3 cup cider vinegar
- 2 teaspoons of fresh dill
- 1 cup water
- 3 whole cloves
- 4 cloves garlic, whole
- 8 whole black peppercorns

- 1/3 teaspoon red pepper flakes
- 8 whole coriander seeds

Directions

1. trim the edges of the asparagus and cut it into lengths.
2. Combine all ingredients in containers that can be airtight.

Nutrition Facts

Servings: 2
Amount per serving
Calories   74
% Daily Value*
Total Fat 0.5g   1%
Saturated Fat 0.1g   1%
Cholesterol 0mg 0%
Sodium 14mg   1%
Total Carbohydrate 14g   5%
Dietary Fiber 5.4g   19%
Total Sugars 5.2g
Protein 5.4g

Marinated Portobello Mushrooms with Provolone

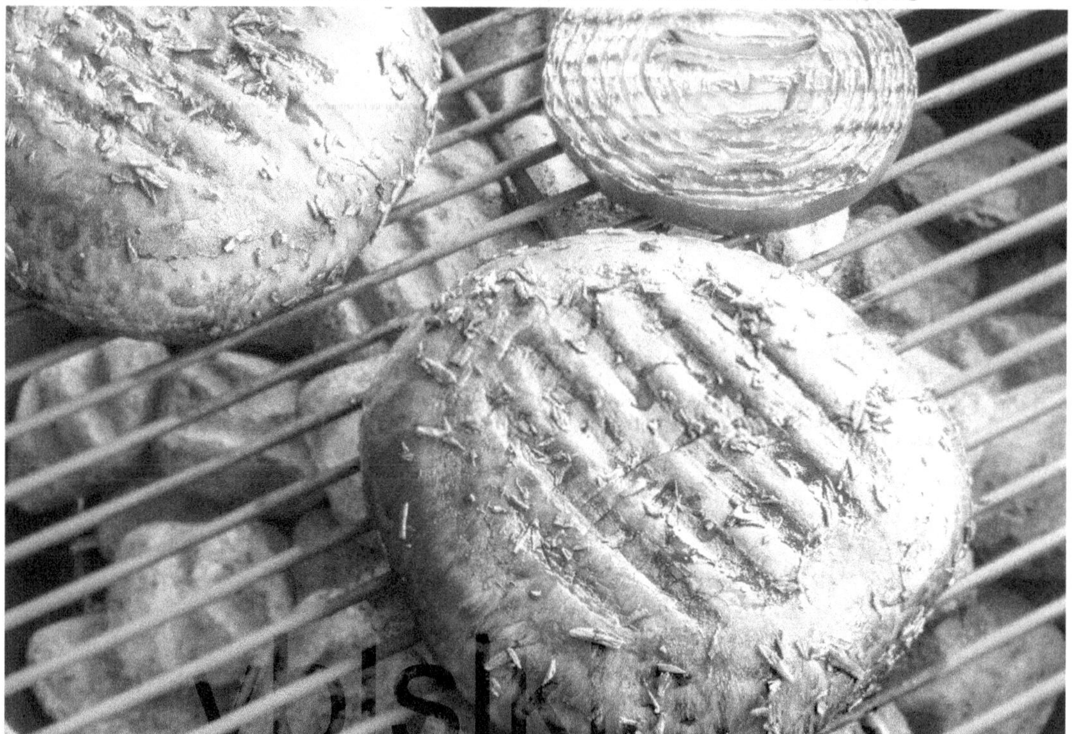

Preparation Time: 15 minutes
Cooking Time: 8 minutes
Servings: 2

Ingredients

- 4 Portobello mushrooms, stemmed and wiped clean
- 1 cup balsamic vinegar
- 2 tablespoons orange juice
- ½ teaspoon dried rosemary
- 2teaspoons minced garlic
- 2 ounces of provolone cheese

Directions

1. First, preheat the grill.

2. Place rack 4 inches above the heat source.
3. Coat the baking tray with cooking oil.
4. Put the mushrooms in the dish, stem less-side up.
5. Whisk the vinegar, orange juice, rosemary, and garlic.
6. pour it over the mushrooms.
7. Grill the mushrooms for 4 minutes on each side.
8. Once it has done add cheese on top.
9. Serve it hot.

Nutrition Facts
Servings: 2
Amount per serving
Calories   157
% Daily Value*
Total Fat 8.4g   11%
Saturated Fat 5.1g   25%
Cholesterol 20mg   7%
Sodium 255mg   11%
Total Carbohydrate 5.1g   2%
Dietary Fiber 1.8g   7%
Total Sugars 2.4g
Protein 10.4g

10 Dinner Recipes

Fish Tacos

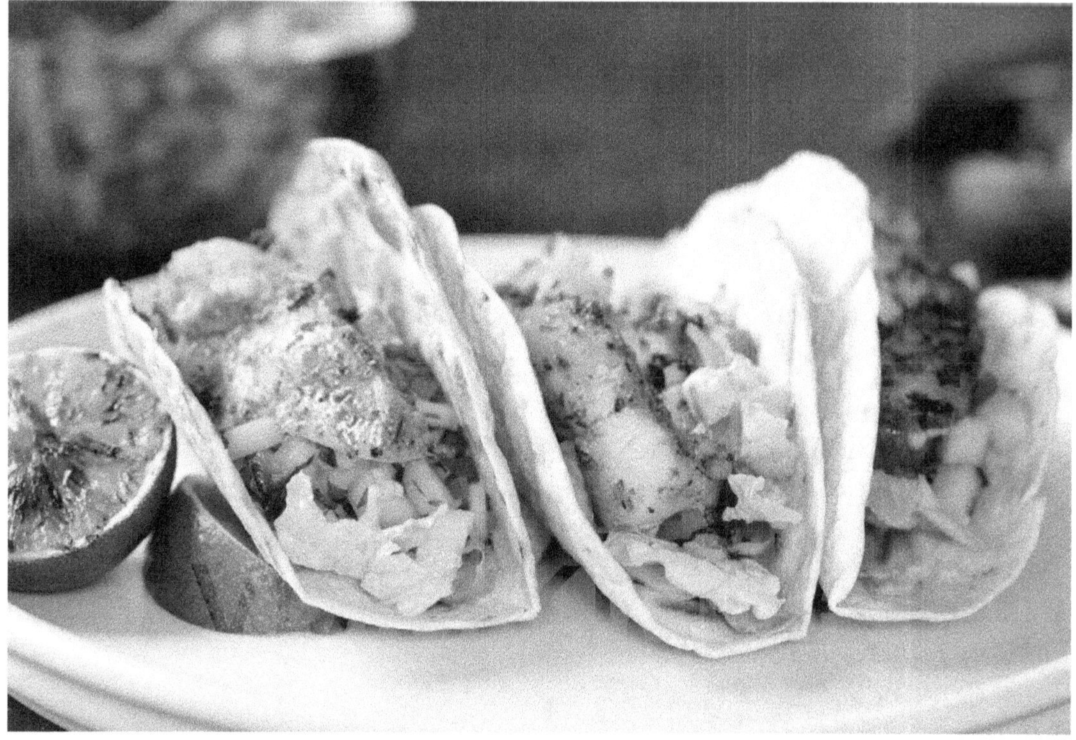

Preparation Time: 15 minutes
Cooking Time: 15 minutes
Servings: 3

Ingredients

- 2 pounds fish fillets
- 2 tablespoons lemon juice
- 2 tomatoes, chopped
- 1 onion, chopped
- 1 tablespoon cilantro, chopped
- 2 teaspoons olive oil
- 1/3 teaspoon cayenne pepper (optional)

- 1/3 teaspoon black pepper
- 6whole wheat tortilla

Directions

1. warm the tortilla wraps in the microwave for a few minutes.
2. next, preheat the oven to 375 degrees F.
3. take a bowl and combine onion, lemon juice, tomato, cilantro, olive oil, cayenne pepper, and black pepper.
4. place this mixture onto fish filets.
5. Bake the fish in preheated oven until it is golden brown for 15-20 minutes.
6. Divide the baked fish among the tortilla wraps and serve.
7. Enjoy.

Nutrition Facts

Servings: 3
Amount per serving
Calories   981
% Daily Value*
Total Fat 42.6g   55%
Saturated Fat 9.1g   45%
Cholesterol 103mg   34%
Sodium 1877mg 82%
Total Carbohydrate 102.4g   37%
Dietary Fiber 9.5g   34%
Total Sugars 3.9g
Protein 53.6g

Spicy Chicken with Broccoli

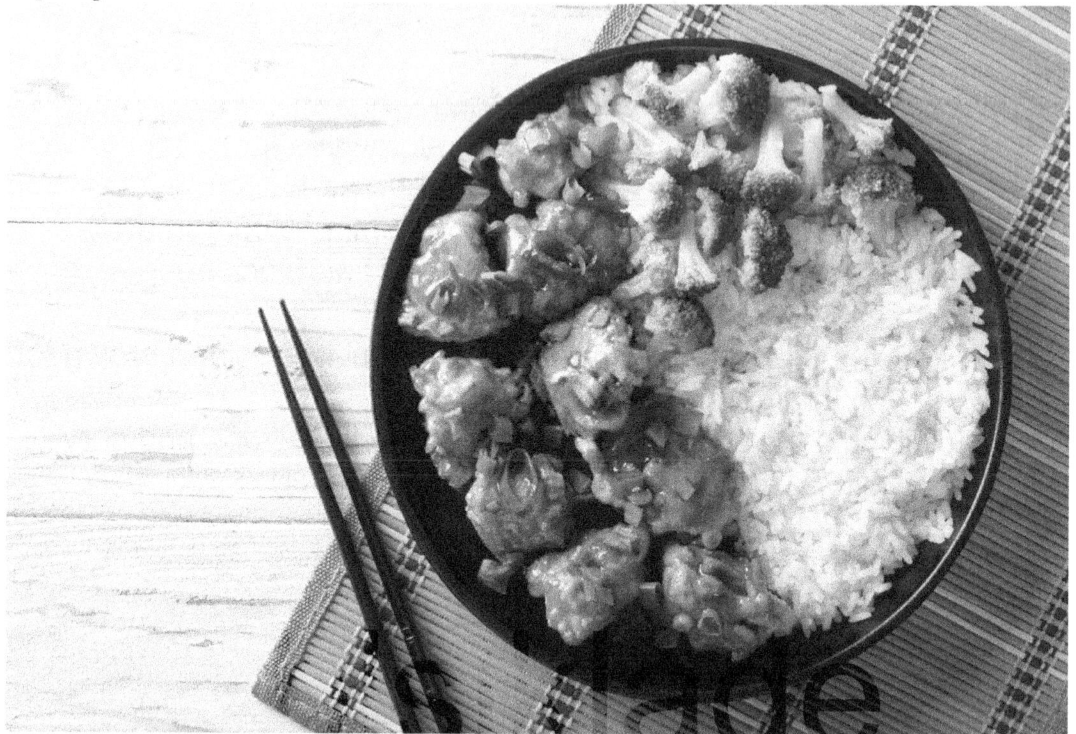

Preparation Time: 15 minutes
Cooking Time: 25 minutes
Servings: 4

Ingredients

- 2.5 pounds of chicken breasts, cut into cubes and boneless
- 2 tablespoons of olive oil
- ½ teaspoon of, Cloves
- 2 teaspoons of fennel seeds
- 2 Star anise
- 1 teaspoon of Ginger, paste
- ¼ teaspoon cayenne pepper
- 2 tablespoons of coconut amino
- 2 green onions, chopped

- 2 cups of broccoli
- 1 cup mushrooms, chopped
- 1 cup water
- 1 tablespoon of cornstarch
- 1 tablespoon of water
- 2 tablespoons of sesame seed
- 2 cups cooked brown rice, optional

Directions

1. Heat half of the oil in a skillet and cook chicken until brown.
2. Then add fennel seeds, star anise, ginger, cayenne pepper, cloves, and coconut amino.
3. Cook for about 2 minutes, and then turn off the heat.
4. Add remaining oil and stir fry the onions, mushrooms, and broccoli in a separate skillet or frying pan.
5. Pour in the half cup of water and chicken15 to the pan.
6. Cook for about 8 minutes.
7. Meanwhile, mix the cornstarch with water.
8. Pour it in as well.
9. Let it cook until thickened.
10. Sprinkle the sesame seeds and serve with steamed rice if liked.

Nutrition Facts

Servings: 4

Amount per serving

Calories   1003

% Daily Value*

Total Fat 33.2g   43%

Saturated Fat 7.6g   38%

Cholesterol 252mg   84%

Sodium 270mg   12%

Total Carbohydrate 80.2g   29%
Dietary Fiber 5.8g   21%
Total Sugars 1.3g
Protein 92.1g

Spinach-Stuffed Chicken

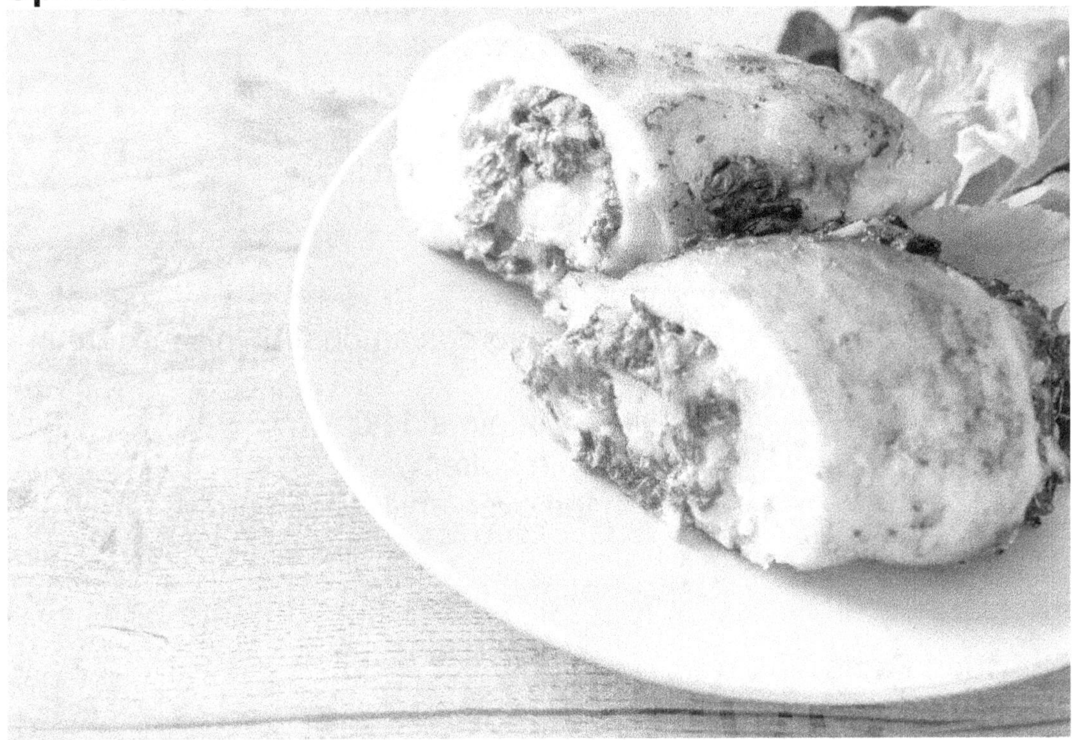

Preparation Time: 15 minutes
Cooking Time: 2o minutes
Servings: 4
Ingredients

2 teaspoons olive oil
2 cups fresh spinach leaves
2 teaspoons of minced garlic
Black pepper, to taste
2 pounds chicken breast pieces, butterfly style cut
1 cup ricotta cheese
3 teaspoons butter, melted
Cooking spray, for greasing

Directions

1. First, wash and pat dry the chicken.
2. use a knife to butterfly cut as it opens like a book.
3. Preheat the oven to 375 degrees F.
4. take a baking dish and grease it with oil spray.
5. take a skillet and heat oil in it.
6. cook spinach, pepper, and garlic in it.
7. Cook it until ingredients get soft.
8. let the ingredients get cool.
9. add in cheese and mix well.
10. place the generous amount of this mixture in the middle chicken breast.
11. Roll breast seam-side down.
12. Brush it with butter.
13. Bake in the oven until golden brown for 20 minutes.
14. Serve hot and enjoy.

Nutrition Facts
Servings: 4
Amount per serving
Calories   480
% Daily Value*
Total Fat 17.2g   22%
Saturated Fat 7.2g   36%
Cholesterol 201mg   67%
Sodium 253mg   11%
Total Carbohydrate 4.2g   2%
Dietary Fiber 0.4g   1%
Total Sugars 0.3g
Protein 73.3g

Thai-Style Chicken

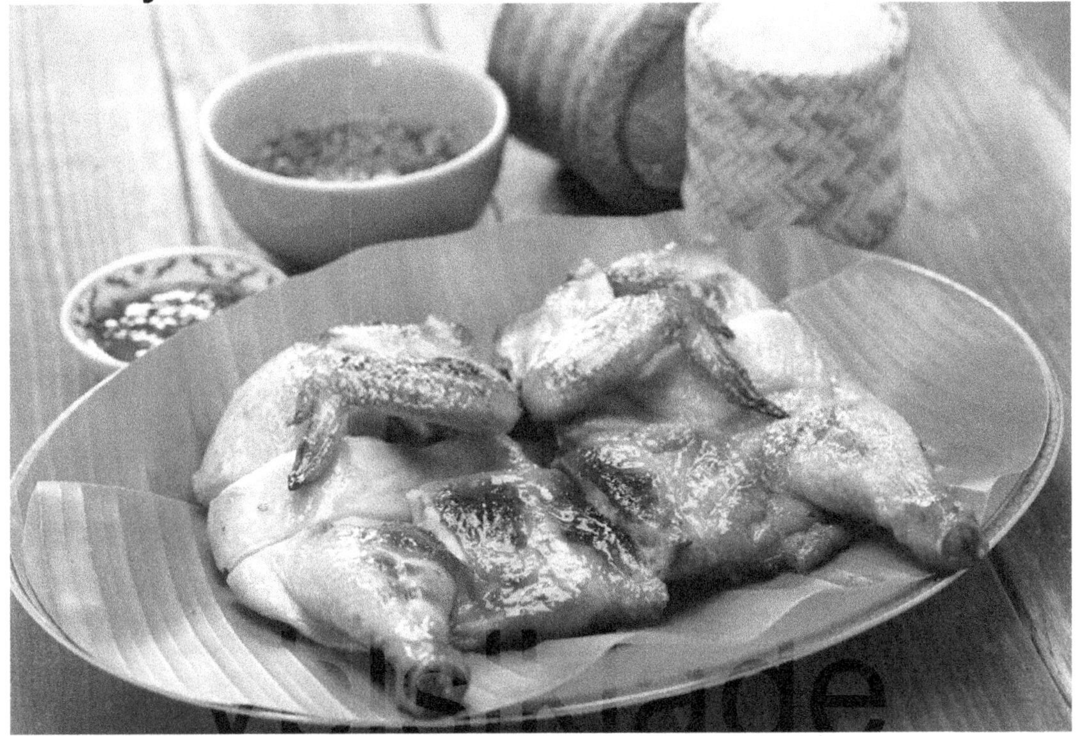

Preparation Time: 15 minutes
Cooking Time: 25 minutes
Servings: 4

Ingredients

- ½ cup peanut Butter
- 1 teaspoon of garlic powder
- ½ teaspoon ginger, ground
- 1 lemon, juice only
- 2 pounds chicken, pieces

Directions

1. Preheat the oven to 400 Degree F.

2. Take a bowl and mix the peanut butter, garlic, ginger, and lemon juice
3. Rub the chicken with it and let it marinate for a few minutes.
4. transfer the chicken to an oil greased tray.
5. Bake in preheated oven for about 25 minutes.
6. Once done serve and enjoy.

Nutrition Facts
Servings: 4
Amount per serving
Calories   539
% Daily Value*
Total Fat 23.2g   30%
Saturated Fat 5.4g   27%
Cholesterol 175mg   58%
Sodium 292mg   13%
Total Carbohydrate 8.4g   3%
Dietary Fiber 2.4g   9%
Total Sugars 3.6g
Protein 74.1g

Celery and Potatoes Recipe

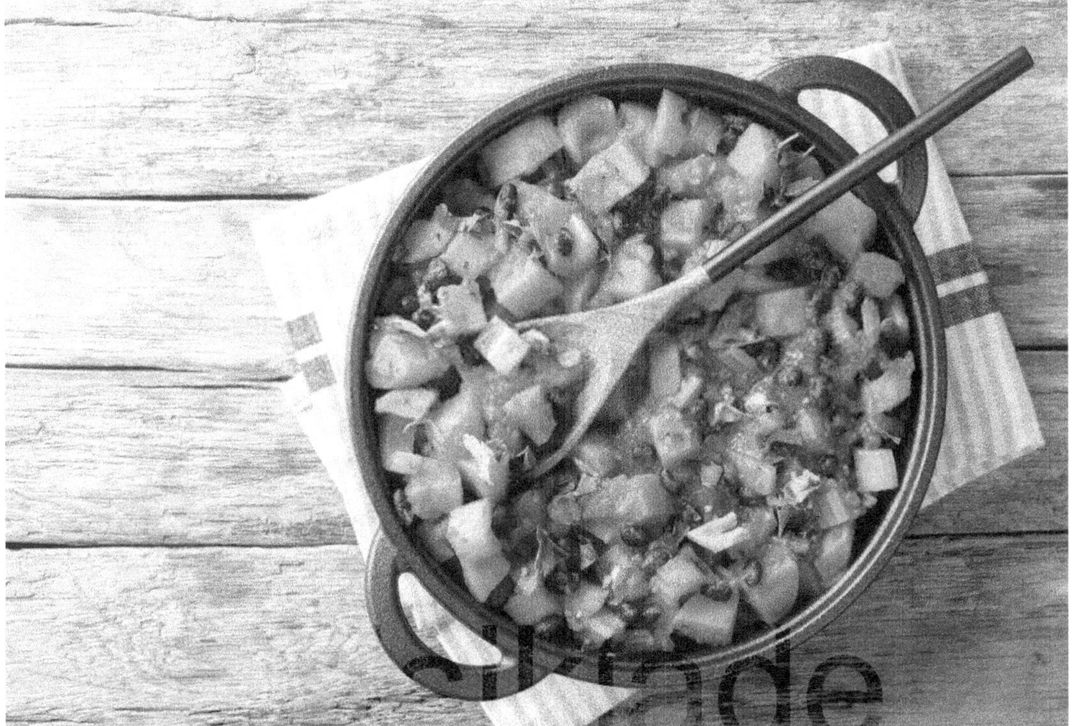

Preparation Time: 15 minutes
Cooking Time: 5 hours 2o minutes
Servings: 2-4

Ingredients

- 4 medium potatoes, peeled and cut into cubes
- 1 cup onion, chopped
- 1 cup carrots, sliced
- 1 cup celery sticks, sliced
- 2 chicken bouillon cubes
- 2 tablespoons parsley flakes
- 6 cups water
- ½ cup olive oil
- 2 cups of milk, low fat

- 2 servings of brown rice, cooked

Directions

1. Put all the ingredients in a slow cooker (excluding milk) and cook on low heat for about 5 hours.
2. After 5 hours, open the pot and pour in the milk.
3. Cook for 20 more minutes and then serve over cooked brown rice.

Nutrition Facts
Servings: 4
Amount per serving
Calories   835
% Daily Value*
Total Fat 28.8g   37%
Saturated Fat 4.2g   21%
Cholesterol 0mg 0%
Sodium 354mg   15%
Total Carbohydrate 133.1g   48%
Dietary Fiber 10.4g   37%
Total Sugars 5.3g
Protein 13.6g

Lentil and Rice Recipe

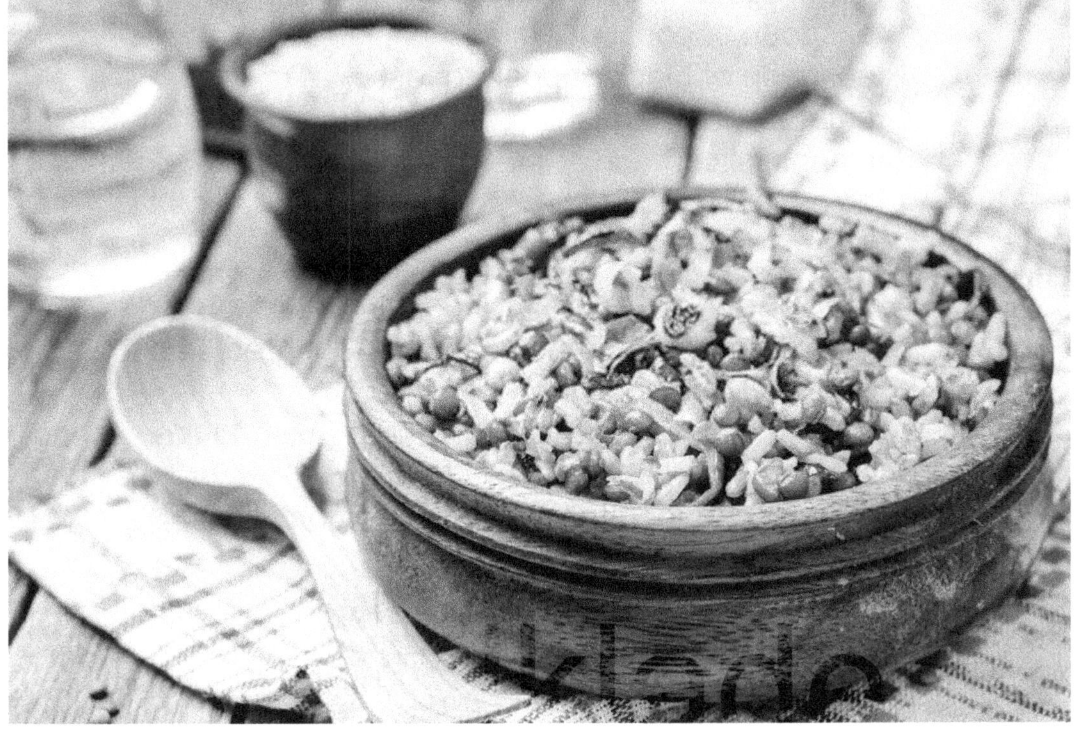

Preparation Time: 15 minutes
Cooking Time: 4 hours
Servings: 6

Ingredients

- 1/3 teaspoon curry powder
- 1 teaspoon cumin, grounded
- 5 large onions, chopped
- 4 cloves garlic, crushed and minced
- 4 cups of spinach, chopped
- 2 teaspoons of ginger, paste
- 2/4 teaspoon turmeric
- 1/1 teaspoon cayenne
- 2 cups lentils, rinsed

- 3 cups rice, rinsed
- 5 cups vegetable broth
- 1 teaspoon of coconut amino
- 1 teaspoon of black pepper, to taste
- 4 tomatoes, for garnishing (chopped)
- 2 lemons, sliced
- 4 tablespoons of butter

Directions

1. Take a Crockpot and add all the listed ingredients to it.
2. Lock the lid and cook for 4 hours.
3. Then turn off the heat and transfer the dish to the serving bowls.
4. Top it with chopped tomatoes and lemon slices.

Nutrition Facts

Servings: 6
Amount per serving
Calories   748
% Daily Value*
Total Fat 10.8g   14%
Saturated Fat 5.5g   28%
Cholesterol 20mg   7%
Sodium 726mg   32%
Total Carbohydrate 132.4g   48%
Dietary Fiber 25.8g   92%
Total Sugars 10.1g
Protein 30.5g

Mexican style bake

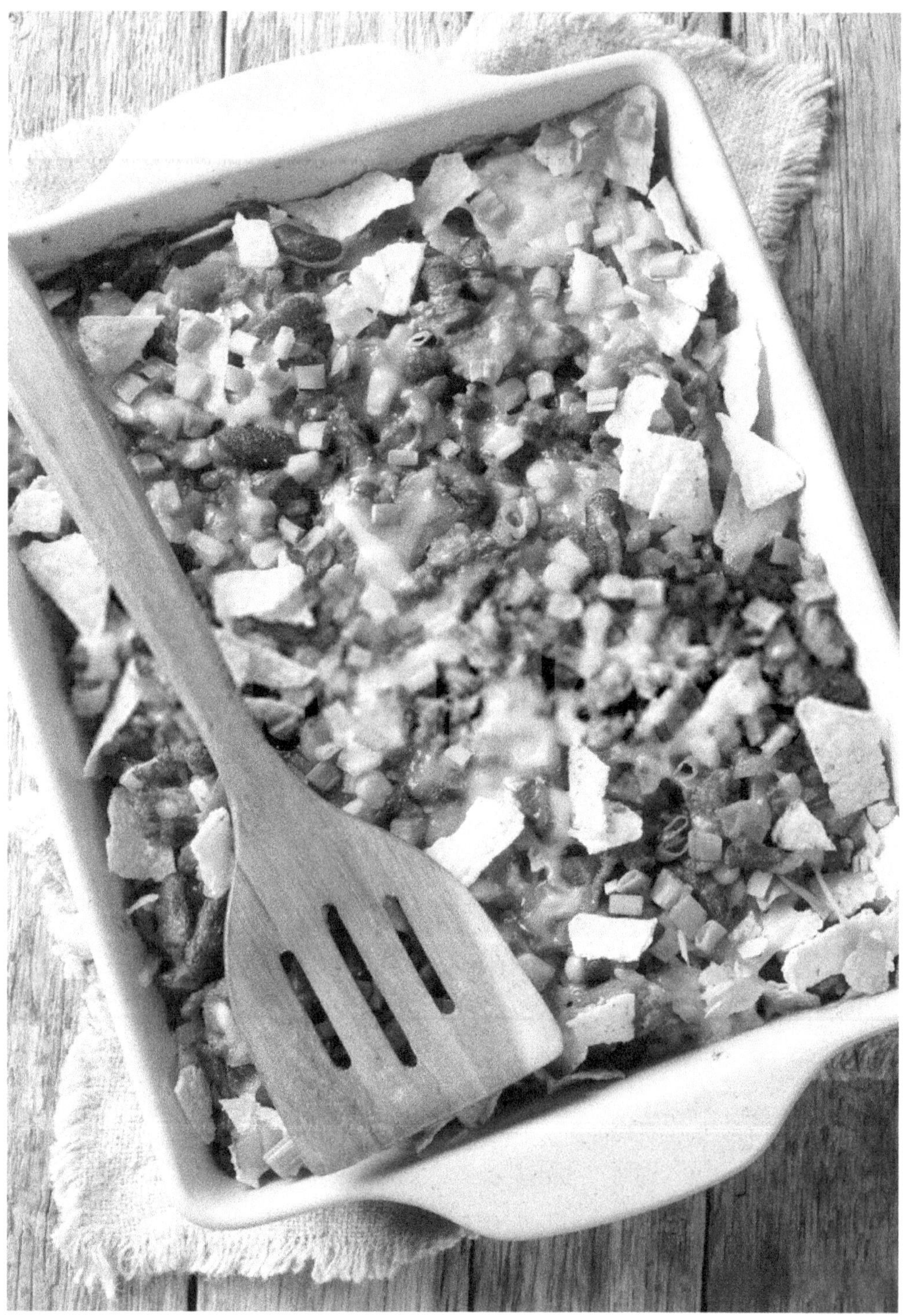

Preparation Time: 25 minutes
Cooking Time: 45 minutes
Servings: 3

Ingredients

- 1.5 cups cooked rice,
- 1 .5-pound skinless, boneless chicken breast cut in bite-sized pieces
- 16 ounces tomatoes, crushed
- 16 ounces black beans, rinsed
- 1-1/4 cup corn kernels
- 1-1/4 cup red bell pepper, cubed
- 1 cup poblano pepper, chopped
- 2 tablespoons chili powder
- 1 tablespoon cumin
- 6 garlic cloves, crushed
- 1 cup Monterey Jack cheese, shredded
- ¼ cup jalapeno pepper, sliced

Directions

1. The first step is to preheat the oven at 400 degrees F.
2. Take a shallow casserole and spread rice on it.
3. Top it with chicken.
4. Then mix chili powder, cumin, garlic cloves, crushed beans, pepper, corn, tomatoes, garlic and pour it over chicken.
5. Top with jalapeno and cheese.
6. Let it bake for 45 minutes.
7. Then serve it.

Nutrition Facts

Servings: 3
Amount per serving

Calories   1227
% Daily Value*
Total Fat 19.3g   25%
Saturated Fat 9.2g   46%
Cholesterol 77mg   26%
Sodium 471mg   20%
Total Carbohydrate 198.4g   72%
Dietary Fiber 30.6g   109%
Total Sugars 14.4g
Protein 71g

Poached Whitefish

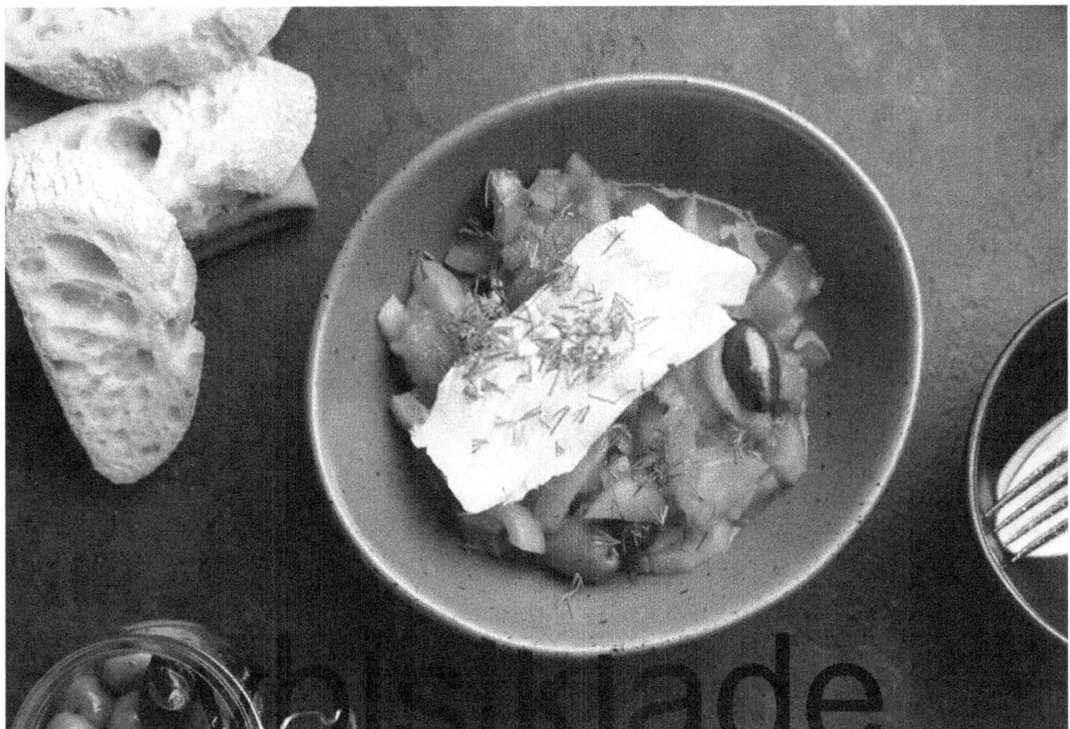

Preparation Time: 15 minutes
Cooking Time: 12 minutes
Servings: 2

Ingredients

- 3 tablespoons of olive oil
- 3 bulbs fennel, chopped
- 1/2 onion, chopped
- 1.5 pounds of whitefish fillets
- 1 pinch saffron
- 3 tablespoons of fennel seeds
- 2 cups of tomatoes, diced
- 1 cup of water

Directions

1. Take a cooking pot and heat oil in it
2. Then saut é onions in it
3. Now add fennel bulbs and stir well.
4. Cook until ingredients are soft
5. Then add tomatoes and saffron
6. Pour in the water and let the boil come
7. Then add fish and fennel seeds
8. Cover and cook for 12 minutes
9. Once it is cooked, serve hot.

Nutrition Facts

Servings: 2
Amount per serving
Calories   501
% Daily Value*
Total Fat 36.3g   47%
Saturated Fat 6.2g   31%
Cholesterol 52mg   17%
Sodium 697mg   30%
Total Carbohydrate 27.5g   10%
Dietary Fiber 6.1g   22%
Total Sugars 5.2g
Protein 22.1g

Lemon-Tahini with Chicken & Vegetables

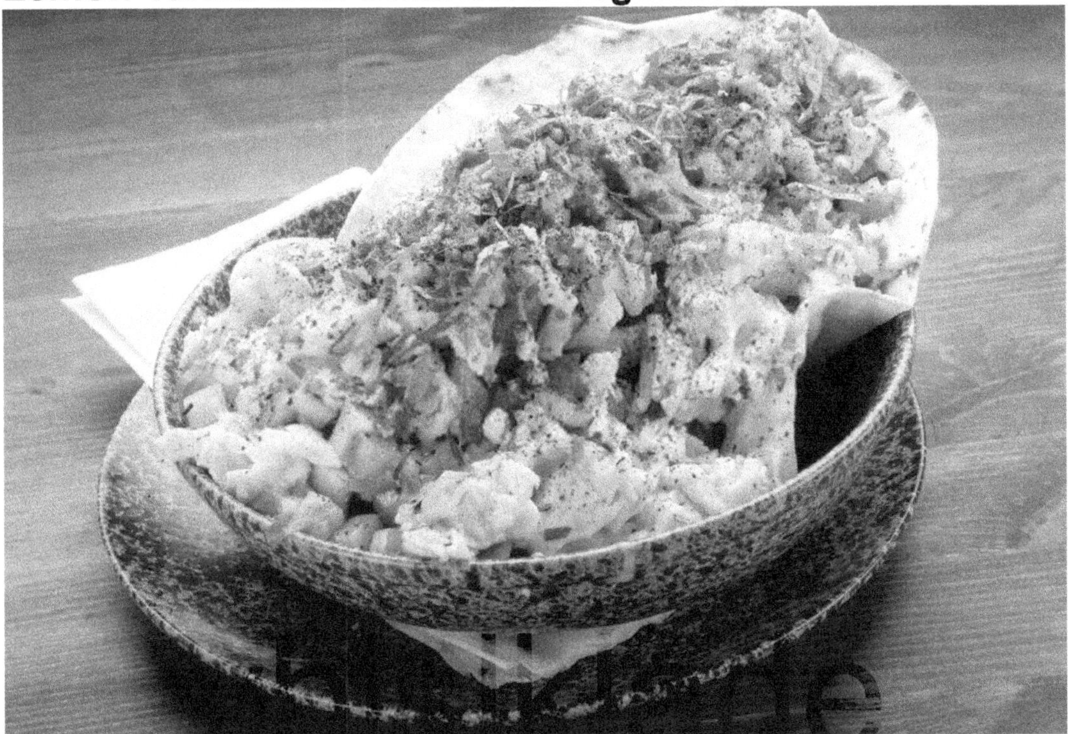

Preparation Time: 15 minutes
Cooking Time: 34 -45 minutes
Servings: 2

Ingredients

- 1.2 cups whole-wheat pearl couscous
- 1/3 cup tahini
- 1/3 teaspoon ground pepper
- 1/3 teaspoon red pepper, crushed
- 2 cloves of garlic, minced
- 2 cups sliced mushrooms
- 1 medium red bell pepper, chopped
- 1/3 cup water
- 2.5 teaspoons lemon zest

- 3.5 cups coleslaw mix
- 3cups baby spinach
- 10 ounces cooked chicken breast, chopped (about 2 1/2 cups)
- 1/3 cup toasted sliced almonds
- 3 tablespoons lemon juice
- 1.5 tablespoons olive oil, divided
- 1/3 cup crumbled reduced-fat feta cheese
- 2 tablespoons chopped fresh parsley
- 1 lemon, cut into wedges

Directions

1. Cook couscous according to package directions.
2. Once done, fluff and set aside.
3. Mix the tahini, lemon juice, pepper, water, half of the oil, and crushed red pepper in a I bowl.
4. Heat the remaining oil in a skillet and cook garlic.
5. then add the mushrooms and the red bell pepper.
6. cook for 3 minutes.
7. Stir in coleslaw mix and spinach/
8. cook for 2 minutes.
9. add the couscous and chicken.
10. then add the tahini sauce; cook for 3-4 minutes.
11. Sprinkle feta, lemon zest, parsley.
12. Serve with lemon wedges.

Nutrition Facts

Servings: 2
Amount per serving
Calories   925
% Daily Value*
Total Fat 51.8g   66%

Saturated Fat 8.9g   44%
Cholesterol 145mg   48%
Sodium 449mg   20%
Total Carbohydrate 64.8g   24%
Dietary Fiber 11.7g   42%
Total Sugars 5.4g
Protein 57g

Creamy Lemon Pasta with Shrimp

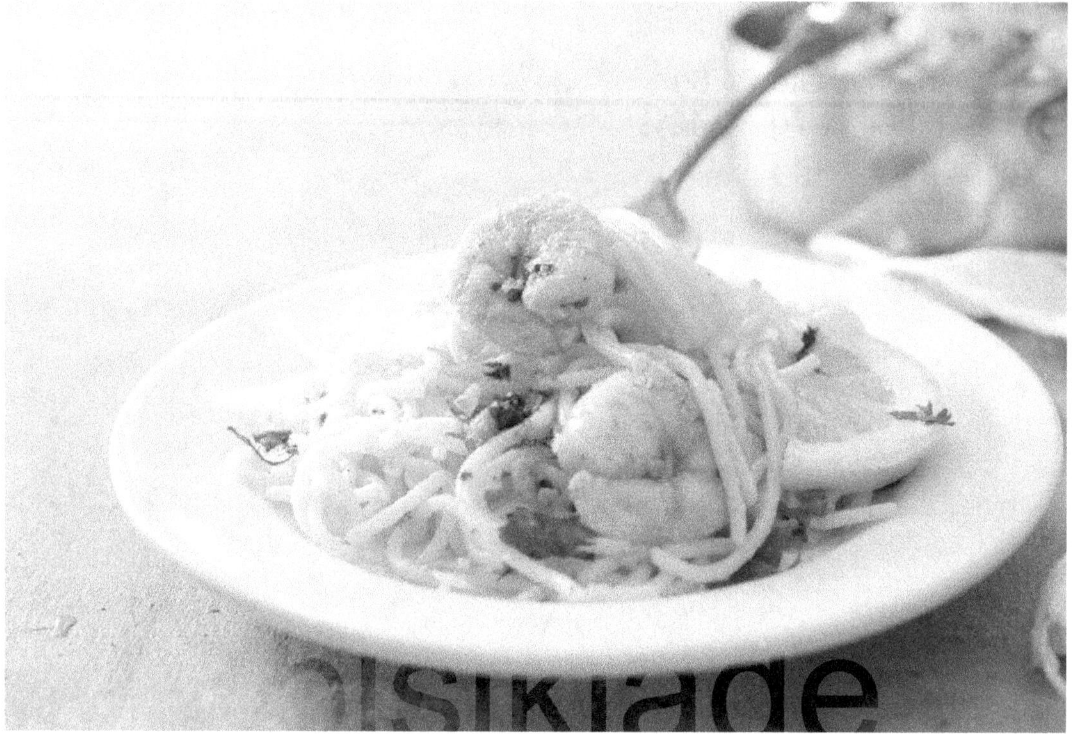

Preparation Time: 15 minutes
Cooking Time: 30 minutes
Servings: 4

Ingredients:

- 7 ounces whole-wheat fettuccine
- 1/3 tablespoon garlic, finely chopped
- 1/3 teaspoon red pepper, crushed
- 2 tablespoons olive oil
- 10 ounces raw shrimp, peeled and deveined
- ¼ cup basil, sliced
- 2 cups arugula, loosely packed
- ¼ cup plain yogurt
- 2 tablespoons butter, unsalted

- 1 teaspoon lemon zest
- 2 tablespoons lemon juice
- 1/3 Cup grated Parmesan cheese

Directions:

1. Take a cooking pot, pour in the water, and let it boil.
2. Then put in the fettuccine.
3. Cook for 10 minutes.
4. Reserve about half a cup of its water and drain.
5. Meanwhile, take a skillet and warm oil.
6. Then put in the shrimp and let it cook for 3 minutes.
7. Drain and set aside.
8. Add the butter to the cooking pan and cook the garlic and crushed red pepper for 1 minute; then add the arugula and let it cook for 2 minutes
9. Then add cooked fettuccine, lemon zest, yogurt, and the reserved pasta water.
10. Next add the lemon juice, shrimp.
11. Toss in parmesan.
12. Top it with basil.
13. Serve.

Nutrition Facts

Servings: 4
Amount per serving
Calories   471
% Daily Value*
Total Fat 20.2g   26%
Saturated Fat 8g 40%
Cholesterol 563mg   188%
Sodium 798mg   35%
Total Carbohydrate 6.2g   2%
Dietary Fiber 0.2g   1%

Total Sugars 0.8g
Protein 63.7g